Herbal Aphrodisiacs
From World Sources

HERBAL APHRODISIACS FROM WORLD SOURCES

including
Anaphrodisiacs
Corrected & Expanded Edition

Compiled, Written & Illustrated by
Clarence Meyer

Meyerbooks, Publisher
Glenwood, Illinois

Cover illustration by Clarence Meyer
Cover by Martin Hertzel Design

Printed on acid-free paper.

Meyerbooks, Publisher
P.O. Box 427
Glenwood, Illinois 60425

TABLE OF CONTENTS

ILLUSTRATIONS

ACKNOWLEDGMENTS

This book would not have been possible without the excellent records of I.H. Burkill, Rev. G.A. Stuart, Dalziel, M.D., J.F. Dastur and authors of earlier times. Credit is extended to informants from Trinidad, Leeward and Winward Islands. Special appreciation is extended to the late Ray Ch. Romain who took the author to his people, to Mambos, Houngans, "leaf docteurs" and through the beautiful mountains of his Haiti.

A NOTE TO THE READER

This book is a record of plants and substances used by races over much of the world, based on the studies of eighty-one authors. Comments without reference to an author are those of the compiler. The compiler and publisher do not recommend the use of any food plants, drug plants, spices or other substances for aphrodisiac and anaphrodisiac purposes without professional medial guidance. Most unfamiliar terms are explained in the Glossary beginning on page 137.

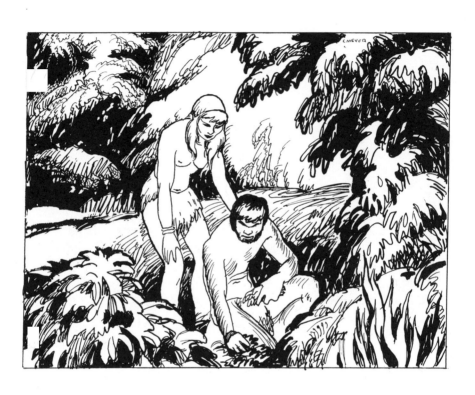

ENDLESS SEARCH

At some remote period of history man was like any other animal: just fortunate to keep alive from day to day. As he developed a safer world for himself he attained an older age and also acquired some disadvantages that generally come with living more years. In youth life is full of pleasures: virile, lusty and almost inexhaustible. Benevolent Nature replenishes the body as fast as youth uses or squanders her gifts.

Virility is the symbol of manhood; it is as important to the male as the crow and strut of the rooster among a flock of hens. The insidious creeping of age, which brings the tendency of developing a cloak of fat, the feeling of little aches and pains, the reduction of activity and the lessening of strength, is so gradual, it goes unheeded until becoming very pronounced. While most changes in the meridian of life go unnoticed, the slightest decline of sexual powers immediately becomes of great concern to the male ego. Mother Nature was good to man in supplying sustenance and medicine for his well being, so it was natural for man to go to her first in the search for a wonder food or drug that would help him retain the sexual cornucopia of youth. As his mental powers increased (with age) he extended his search into the earth and seas, made mixtures and eventually stumbled into alchemy.

Much of man's earthly accumulations are diverted to sensual

pleasures and the search to increase as well as retain them. As he adds more years to life the search becomes more intensified. Nothing is too good or too bad for his stomach if it gives him a measure of youth and pleasure. He is willing to undergo tortures for magic results. Eating insects, horns, hoofs, offal, embryos, placenta, morbid secretions and virulent poisons from plants, earth and seas reveals Homo sapiens' perseverance. His gullibility is ridiculously exposed when alchemists convinced the aging and dissipated to believe that "potable" gold introduced into the animal system would provide an inexhaustible source of strength and virility. Throughout the ages rare, exotic and costly ingredients, including pearls and gems, were added to concoctions to "enhance their properties" and to increase their shekel value. Conquerors, despots, kings, the titular, and the wealthy were usually the most gullible of virility seekers. They enjoyed the pleasures of life and did not want to give them up even after Nature had already provided them with all or more than their due for the normal span of the human species.

New and strange plants invariably kindled fresh hope for rejuvenation and longer life. When Marco Polo and early traders brought spices from the Far East, their exhilarating aromas and flavors were at once acclaimed sex stimulants. An early seventeenth century recipe states: "The weight of foure drams of the pouder of Cloves taken in milke procureth the act of generation." *The Family Companion for Health* (1730) gives the following: "Cloves are of good Use for decay'd Venery, by taking their Powder to some handsome quantity in Sack once or twice a Day: Thus the aged and jaded Constitution often have Recourse to Cantharides to produce this Effect, and hazard their lives by it; whereas these may be taken in pretty large Quantity, and no ill consequences will ensu, and they have been confess'd of use by many."

Spices were particularly held in high esteem in the Orient. In Mohammedan medicine, nutmeg and mace were believed to be stimulant, digestive, tonic as well as aphrodisiacs. Cinnamon was believed capable of inspiring love; its use as an aphrodisiac is mentioned in early Persian literature. Familiarity with spices eventually wore off aphrodisiac notions in the Western World and spices were used merely to arouse jaded taste buds or to disguise odors and flavors of foods, medicines and aphrodisiac concoctions.

When the New World was discovered, explorers brought back many strange fruits, vegetables, and medicinal botanicals with fanciful stories associated with their unusual products. The great herbals of Dodoens, Parkinson and Gerarde provided more detailed information on New World plants than earlier records, which expressed more amazement at the new wonders than earthy facts. Gerarde wrote regarding the Flower of the Sun, our common sunflower: "The buds, before they be floured, boiled and eaten with butter, vinegar, and pepper, after the manner of Artichokes, are exceeding pleasant meat [food], surpassing the Artichoke far in procuring bodily lust. The same buds with the stalks neere unto the top (the hairinesse being taken away) broiled upon a gridiron, and after eaten with oile, vinegar, and pepper, have the like properties."

The potato, food of the Incas, was also exploited as an aphrodisiac in the early days of its introduction to Europe. Parkinson mentioned: "The Comfit-makers preserve them and candy them as divers other things, and so ordered, is very delicate, fit to accompany such other banquetting dishes."

Gerarde wrote of another introduction from the New World. "Notwithstanding howsoever they [sweet potato] are dressed, they comfort, nourish, and strengthen the body, vehemently procuring bodily lust." The sweet potato was also known in Gerarde's time as Skyrrets of Peru, because of their slight similarity to a popular aphrodisiac (skirrets) much used in old Europe.

Europeans were very apprehensive of the tomato for more than a century after it was introduced. Dodoens description of Amorus Apples [tomato] is interesting. He cautioned - "All the herbe is of a strange stinking savour.... The complexion, nature, and working of this plant is not yet knowne, but by that I can gather of the

3

taste, it should be colde of nature, especially the leaves, somewhat like unto Mandrake, and therefore also it is dangerous to be used." In 1722 Joseph Miller added medicinal uses to Amoris Pomum or Apples of love. "They [tomatoes] are seldom eaten with us, being of the Nature of the other Solanums; and therefore only used outwardly in cooling and moistening applications, in Inflammations and Erysipelas; and its Juice especially is commended in hot Defluxions of Rheum upon the Eyes. It is but seldom used."

The luscious tomato - poisonous or not - was too tempting for the Italians. They learned to eat them with vinegar, garlic, olive oil and salt. Travelers noted how avidly the Apples of Love were eaten and apparently assumed that they contributed much to the Italian male's Casanova-like nature. The travelers took their beliefs and perhaps spiced the stories a bit for greater impression upon folks at home. Soon after most of Europe was growing and eating tomatoes.

Chocolate (*Theobroma cacao*), vanilla and other New World products also were considered aphrodisiacs. Gerarde thought bananas "stirreth to generation" and wrote there were some who judged it to be the forbidden fruit and believed it to be the original Adam's Apple tree.

Most famous of all searchers for the Fountain of Youth was Juan Ponce de Leon. He was in his early 50s while governor of Puerto Rico and immensely enjoyed all the pleasures of life. Like most successful men, he wanted to prolong these pleasures, and at his age the vigor for enjoyments was not increasing. If Juan over-indulged, as one generally does when so much is available, his powers were most likely waning and becoming a concern.

Indians of the Caribbean held many legends, and those associated with gold or rejuvenation were of particular interest to the Spaniards. The legend of the Fountain of Youth was of special attraction to Juan Ponce de Leon. According to history he sailed from Santa Domingo, the capital of Spanish New World, in 1513 to seek the mythical spring of virility and rejuvenation. The search took Juan to a strange land with vast areas of razor-edged grass in

4

which grew scattered hammock jungles and, in lower lands, groves of stumpy swamp palms. In the upper ground levels long-needle pine trees stood high above impenetrable saw-palmetto. Juan saw this new land shortly after a rainy spell which brought forth a profusion of spring flowers. For this reason his new discovery was named Florida, or the land of flowers. It is doubtful Juan ever saw the unique crystal clear springs in northern Florida. They probably would have been mistaken for the mythical springs if one was exhausted, covered with insects, bruises and scratches from torturous traveling in wilderness under a searing Florida sun.

About 200 years after Ponce de Leon's search, Father Lafitau discovered in the northern forests of the New World a plant that remarkably fit the description of a wondrous herb of China. The Father must have been deeply impressed with his discovery because he had read the report and personal experiences of Father Jartoux, a brother missionary in China. The wondrous herb of china was known as jenshen or ginseng. For more than 5,000 years ginseng was extolled as a panacea for all ills. Reverend Stuart wrote the root of this plant was, "the dernier ressort when all other drugs fail." Chinese physicians wrote volumes upon ginseng's virtues, and no medicine was thought to be of any value unless it contained a portion of ginseng. Berdoe mentioned when a Chinese physician is not able to procure the medicines he needs, he writes the names of the drugs he desires to employ on a piece of paper, and makes the patient swallow it. The effect is supposed to be quite as good as that of the remedy itself. Without a doubt many poor patients that could not afford the root reserved for emperors and mandarins had to swallow the paper on which jen-shen was written.

Gardens Bulletin (1930) states, "The best ginseng formerly came from the Kirin province of Manchuria, the cultivation and collection being a government monopoly, but the supply is now very rare. Korean ginseng is regarded as the best, but it is frequently adulterated with roots of other plants." The demand for ginseng in the Orient far exceeded the supply, and Stuart's book

5

Chinese Materia Medica (1911), names eight fraudulent substitutes and adds other roots were also substituted. [See *Panax ginseng, P. quinquefolia* and *Sium sisarum.*] Crafty dealers resorted to skillful flavoring and coloring treatments, soaking roots in rice water and steam-curing with millet seed in order to make entirely unrelated roots look and taste like the genuine article.

Father Lafitau's American plant was a perfect substitute for the extremely rare and costly Chinese ginseng. The American species was, moreover, very common in a large range extending along the Atlantic from northern Florida into Canada and westward in much of the wilderness extending to the Great Lakes. Gunn's *Domestic Medicine* (1834) states: "It [ginseng] is found in great plenty among the hills and mountains of Tennessee." Bowker's *Indian Vegetable Family Instructor* (1836) adds: "This root abounds in great plenty throughout the woods and fields of Vermont." American ginseng became a bonanza for pioneers, fur traders, Indians and anyone that knew the plant. George Washington wrote in his diary after a visit to Ohio in 1784: "In passing over the Mountains, I met numbers of Persons and Pack horses going in with Ginseng." Daniel Boone gathered ginseng in Kentucky and took the roots up the Ohio River to ship to Philadelphia. Fortunes were made and the trade with the Orient was a windfall for America's infant maritime fleet.

When American ginseng was brought to China, dealers again devised a way to make the New World plant look like their panacea. *Gardens Bulletin* reveals, "The roots are made to resemble the Chinese drug by freeing them from their epidermis, and making what is called in the Customs, 'clarified' ginseng." The once prolific American ginseng now is nearly grubbed to extinction in the wild state, and like the Oriental plant must be grown on special farms. A quaint picture in *Life in Corea* [Korea] shows a guard on a mounted platform protecting his precious crop of ginseng. The guard has a long watch as the plant requires six years to mature. American ginseng matures in the same number of years.

6

Early explorers of the New World brought back more than new products and aphrodisiacs according to *Joyfull Newes Out of The Newe Founde Worlde* by Nicholes Monardes. The physician from Seville, Spain, gave the following account in 1577:

In the yere of our Lorde God 1493, in the wars that the Catholic king had in Naples, with King Charles of Fraunce, that was called greate heade: in this tyme sir Christofer Colon [Columbus], came from the discoverie that he had made in the Indias. He brought a greate number of Indians, bothe men and women, which he carried with him to Naples, where the Catholic King was at that tyme, who had then concluded the wars, for that there was peace between the two Kings, and the hostes did communicate together, the one with the other. And Colon being come thether with his Indians, the most part of them went with the fruite of their countrie which was the Poxe (syphilis) the Spaniards began to have conversation with the Indian women, in such sorte, that the men and women of the Indias, did infecte the Campe of the Spaniards, Italians and Almaines [Germans], the Catholic king had then of all these Nations, and there were many that was infected of the evill. And after the hostes did common together, the fire did kindle in the camp of the king of Fraunce: of the which did follow that in short tyme, the one and the other were infected to this evill seed: and from thence it hath spred abroad into all the worlde.

At the beginning it had diverse names: the Spaniards did think that it had been given them by the Frenche men, and they called it the Frenche evill. The Frenche men thought that in Naples, and of them of the countrie, the evill had been given them, and they called it the evill of Naples. And they of Almaine seyng that of the conversation of the Spaniards, they came to it, they called it the Spanishe Skabbe, and other called it the Measelles of the Indias, and with much truth, seyng that from thence came the evill.

Whether syphilis originated in the New World or not, ethnobotany records of the American Indians contain more plants used to cure or mitigate venereal diseases than all other records. Indians, of course, could have sought plant remedies after contact with early explorers.

Procreation or sexual drive differs with races as well as individuals; nevertheless sex stimulants or rejuvenators appear to be important to most races. It is interesting that oriental records contain far more botanicals and animal substances thought to be aphrodisiacs than similar records of Europe or of the aboriginal races of the world. Dr. K.M. Nadkarni's (East) *Indian Materia Medica* (1950 ed.), lists more than 90 aphrodisiacs. It is perhaps a coincidence that China and India are the most densely populated regions of the world. Africans had many aphrodisiacs; however, many were mere charms.

American Indians appear to have been least concerned with sex stimulating plants according to ethnobotany records. The aphrodisiac claims of Indian foods brought to Europe apparently were made by traders and soldiers of fortune who wished to turn their discoveries to gold. Sir Walter Raleigh took timely advantage of the frenzy over New World products by shipping many boat loads of a flavorous "wonder drug" called sassafras to Europe. The aphrodisiac claims of cocaine, Muira-puama, Damiana and other botanicals probably originated from Spanish sources.

The mode of the life of American Indians had much to do with their disinterest in sex stimulants. To survive, most tribes had to hunt constantly for food, and the healthy sport kept them physically fit as well as capable of enduring many hardships. Life in the wilderness would not tolerate detrimental health habits and obesity was unheard of among Indians. Simple living and a diet of many wild plants also contributed much to the Indian's stamina and survival. Wild plants are far richer in essentials of diet than our calorie-fattened cultivated plants. One of the earliest reports on the health of the Indians was made by Lahontan in the seventeenth century. He said, "The Savages are very healthy, and unacquainted with an infinity of Diseases that plague the Europeans, such as the Palsey, the Dropsey, the Gout, the Phthisick, the Asthma, the Gravel, and the Stone. . . .Their Victuals are either boiled or roasted, and they lap great quantities of the Broth, both of Meat and of Fish: They cannot bear the taste of Salt or Spices, and wonder that we are able to live so long as thirty years, considering our Wines, our Spices, and our Immoderate Use of Women."

Sophisticated life breeds more thoughts of sex through luxurious living, more idleness and diets overloaded with the richest foods gleaned over the world. Lahontan's remark regarding the white man's "immoderate Use of Women" is particularly interesting. Indians did not know that the civilized world was no longer a man's world. Females had become aware of the potentials of their physical attractions and for thousands of years were using their charms to seduce and subdue the once domineering male.

Procreation has become very complex in modern civilization, and sex drive is channeled into a confusing maze. Perhaps the most common of all deviations is the drive of many business men who use their energies to further their goals over fellow men. Their sex urge is relieved with almost the finesse of a burp. Mutual orgasm is completely forgotten. This self-centered type of male generally seeks and needs aphrodisiacs. Many successful men use their worldly gains to pamper their organs of survival (bellies) with the finest wines, liqueurs and delicacies of the earth and seas. Aphrodisiac foods naturally are part of their sumptuous diet; however, in these types sexual senses are eventually stifled by fat.

Intellectuals often do not enjoy a normal a sex life because their minds are completely absorbed most of twenty-four hours per day with their work, allowing little or no time for simple animal functions. An excellent example was made by Davenport:

A celebrated mathematician of a very robust constitution, having married a young and pretty woman, lived several years with her, but had not the happiness of becoming a father. Far from being insensible to the charms of his fair wife, he, on the contrary, felt frequently impelled to gratify

9

his passion, but the conjugal act, complete in every other respect, was never crowned by the emission of the seminal fluid. The interval of time which occurred between the commencement of his labor of love and the end was always sufficiently long to allow his mind, which had been for a moment abstracted by his pleasure, to be brought back to the constant object of his meditation -- that is, to geometrical problems or algebraical formula. At the very moment even of the orgasm, the intellectual powers resumed their empire and all genital sensation vanished. Peirible, his medical advisor, recommended (to his wife) never to suffer the attentions of her husband until he was, 'half-seas-over,' this appearing to him the only practical means of withdrawing her learned spouse from the influence of the divine Urania and subjecting him more immediately to that of the seductive goddess of Paphos. The advice proved judicious.

Nature endows most individuals, according to heritage, their share of vital forces to perform functions necessary for procreation. Some humans build stronger bloodline by improved living and mating while others will weaken their links by indulging abnormally in pleasures of the senses. Aphrodisiacs may prove useful, but one must pay for immoderate excesses of any kind. Dr. Venner's warning in the year 1650 may appear old-fashioned and obsolete by modern terms, but the basic truth will always remain. The venerable doctor from the town of Bathe, England, advised:

I would have all such as are intemperately addicted to *Venus* (or Aphrodite), to take notice, unless they desire to have their bodies and strengths wasted, spirits consumed, old age and death hastened. For the genital seed, the oyle of life, and comforter of Nature, being a substance full of spirit, which if wilfully wasted, hurteth the body more, than if forty times as much blood were shed or lost. Where those that are of a melancholick, or dry cholerick constitution, must be most wary; for such are soonest, and that very quickly, hurt by *Venus*.

10

PLANTS USED AS APHRODISIACS

A summary of the plants used as aphrodisiacs presents a curious assortment of beliefs as to why they were used for that particular purpose. Little is known about some plants in this book and perhaps what is known will always be regarded as simple folklore. The use of ginseng as an aphrodisiac has continued for 50 centuries or more, and properties attributed to it have not diminished in time. Like many of our official drugs, ginseng has been steeped in mythology. It is incredible that a botanical could be regarded so highly by the world's oldest civilization for so many centuries merely because some roots resemble the body of man. Ginseng may have a more definite action upon the Chinese than Caucasians because of their significant difference in body chemistry. Since remote times Chinese diet consisted mainly of vegetables and rice, while flesh foods have long been used in the diet of Caucasians. Drug habituation, saturations of caffeine, nicotine, alcohol, chemicals in water and foods also may be important factors in affecting the action of a botanical, especially when such a plant has a reputation for gentle properties.

Exhaustive researches have been made on poisonous and powerful acting plants, and when analytical methods become more sophisticated, perhaps the plants tossed aside as old wives' tales or witches' brew will reveal more subtle and elusive atoms or elements that were once thought of no value. Only in recent times was it realized that the insignificant trace elements in the soils had a profound effect upon plants and animals that fed on them. In 1953 only seven trace elements were thought to be essential to animal economy. In 1966 a dozen or so trace elements were known. Today there are fifty known trace elements. Other micronutrient elements in plants may not be important in themselves, yet may be essential to the complex catalytic reactions of metabolism. The lack of trace elements in plants usually is obvious, but the lack of the infinitesimal is far more difficult to discover in humans because of gradual and subtle accumulation over a longer span of life.

Long before vitamins and minerals were isolated and labeled, people knew the foods and plants that gave them more energy than others. A number of plant seeds were used as aphrodisiacs and we now know they are rich in vitamin E, an essential factor for reproduction. B-vitamins, protein carbohydrates, fats and oils, magnesium, phosphorus, calcium and trace elements are also found in seeds. Modern European authorities credit old-time aphrodisiacs, watercress, parsley, tomato, nettles and others as unusually rich sources of vitamins and minerals. Avocado, mustard, onions, garlic, leeks and other *Allium* species are particularly rich in organic sulphur. Powerful metabolic properties are ascribed to calamus, wormwood and stinging nettle by German sources.

Many plants used as aphrodisiacs were simple tonics when general well-being was expected to restore the normal functions of nature.

Mucilaginous plants, such as okra, mallows, *Bombax* and *Orchis* species were used as aphrodisiacs merely because it was believed their jell-like constituent enriched semen. Bland mucilaginous plants (demulcents) are valuable therapeutics used to coat, protect or lubricate delicate mucous membrane passages, allowing inherent healing powers to restore normal conditions. Some roots and fruits regarded as aphrodisiacs contain unusual amounts of saccharin

12

constituents. Licorice root, one of the most ancient of all aphrodisiacs, contains a substance known as glycrrhizin, which is said to
be fifty times sweeter than cane sugar. Licorice is mentioned in
practically all botanical materia medica records throughout man's
history. A generous supply of the root was found in the 3,000
year-old tomb of King Tutankahamen stored with jewelry, and
household goods. The ancient Egyptians believed in life after
death so all the necessities were provided in the tomb. Licorice
certainly was not in the Pharoah's hoard merely for flavoring purposes.

The peculiar sweetish roots of eryngos, calamus and skirret were
once prepared as comfits in Old Europe. Other sweetish botanicals
are candied in the Orient.

In Haiti, the author sampled a peasant liqueur said to be a
powerful aphrodisiac. It tasted much like sugar syrup with a little
vanilla and a good portion of native rum. Brillat-Savarin has
special recipes for amorous excesses which began with heavily
sugared water.

In a recent trip to Germany the author found a "Sex-zucker"
being advertised in popular magazines.

The translation of the advertisement reads:

This new Sex-Sugar works fast. It quickly increases the
sexual lust of women. Unleashes erotic assaults. Quickens
the readiness for love as never before! Can be mixed with
all beverages.

Sugar is reputed to give quick energy--and heat too.

Muira-puama, yohimbe, vitamin E, kola nut, ignatius bean and
ginseng are also prominently advertised in Germany in various
forms for "mehr gluckliche; mehr junge; vorzeitiges Altern;
Leitungsabfall; vitalitat aus der Natur; Lebensaktivator." A
Muira-Puama-Pulver fur Frauen is a special formula available for
ladies.

In 1956, 1957 and 1958 an aphrodisiac (*Rhynchosia*), from the
West Indies was given much publicity by the news media, radio
and magazine articles reviving hope for aging and debilitated

13

males. Hopes were shattered when the Food and Drug Administration stopped the import of the vine.

In the 1930s durian fruit was brought to Germany and then to the United States in the form of pills, confection and marmalades. The first paragraph of the promoter's advertising pamphlet began: "Do you want to learn how to avert physical breakdown and premature old age? How to keep your body vigorous and tireless... your faculties undimmed...your mind alert...your spirit youthful? Do you want your appearance to reflect this physical well being, to have clear, bright eyes, soft, elastic skin, abundant, healthy hair, erect carriage?" This was a circuitous way of saying the product was an aphrodisiac. The pamphlet included an impressive list of European scientists, professors, doctors and clinical reports corroborating the virtues of durian fruit. The wonderful claims were not approved by American authorities and the product went into Limbo with *Rhynchosia*, sarsaparilla, damiana, hydrocotyle, Spanish flies, mandragora and many other "great discoveries" of the past.

Aphrodisiacs are not panaceas that will cure organic or multiple conditions such as hereditary impotence, all nutritional deficiencies, psychological and nervous problems, self-abuse, and normal senility. The search for such a magic cure will continue as long as man retains the natural principle he was endowed with.

APHRODISIACS

Agents which stimulate the sexual appetite and function by direct or reflex action on the genital centers in the brain and spinal cord.

Abrus precatorius: Jequirity, prayer seeds, crab's eyes, wild licorice, jumbi seeds

The seeds contain abrin, a protein toxic, and abric acid and in large doses they are more poisonous than strychnine. The seeds lose their medicinal properties when boiled. The powdered seeds boiled with milk are used as a powerful tonic (in India) and have an aphrodisiacal action on the nervous system, the dose being one to three grains of powder.   Dastur

Ingestion of one jequirity seed has caused fatal poisoning when thoroughly chewed. Nadkarni wrote: "Like all albuminous seeds it loses its activity when boiled, and if administered uncooked they act as strong purgative and emetic; in large doses they are acrid poison, giving rise to symptoms like those of cholera." Safford adds: "It (abrin) is easily decomposed by heat, and in Egypt the seeds are sometimes cooked and eaten when food is scarce, though they are very hard and indigestible."

In India the seeds are ground to powder in a mortar, into which natives dip the points of their daggers, and the wounds inflicted by daggers thus prepared cause death.

Abutilon indicum: Indian mallow

The leaves are reputed to be aphrodisiac. They contain mucilage, tannin, organic acid and traces of asparagin. The ash contains alkaline sulphates, chlorides, magnesium and calcium carbonate. Nadkarni

Abyssinian tea. (See Catha edulis)

Acacia arabica: Babul tree

Fried in ghee, the gum is useful as a nutritive tonic and aphrodisiac in cases of sexual debility. The gum contains arabic acid combined with calcium, magnesium and potassium: also small quantities of malic acid, sugar, moisture (14 percent), and ash (3/4 percent). Nadkarni

Dastur stated that the gum was made into a confection with ghee, sugar and spices. Babul gum is used much like official Acacia.

Acorus calamus: Calamus, sweet flag

The powder thereof drunke, augmenteth seed of generation.
Langham, 1633

Persians and Arabians believe the root increases sexual potency. For sexual weakness of men, drink the infusion of calamus two or three times a day. Rogler

A more recent German source claims early stages of sexual disturbances in men may be cured by drinking for ten days 1/4 liter of cider in which 20 grams calamus has been steeped.

Adenanthera pavonina: Bead tree

A decoction of the leaves or bark, used for a long time, acts as an aphrodisiac. Nadkarni

18

Aframomum melegueta: Grains of Paradise

Seeds said to be used in Africa to disguise poison or drugs administered furtively, such as aphrodisiacs and abortifacients, or to delay their action so as to avert suspicion.   Dalziel

Grains of Paradise were formerly used as a spice and a substitute for black pepper.   The seeds are also used to flavor liqueurs.   Formerly used in England to impart a fictitious appearance of strength to malt and spirituous liquors.

Alchornea floribunda

In the Belgian Congo the plant is know as niando, and the root has been found to have properties similar to those of Indian hemp. The root-bark, dried, pulverized and mixed with food, causes a sort of intoxication, in some cases mild, in others violent, and is made use of to induce a desired temporary excitement or vigor, physical or verbal, and for an aphrodisiac effect.   Or the root-fibres are macerated for several days in palm wine or banana wine, and the liquid is drunk to stimulate energy and excitement in festive dances, etc., often leading to abandoned excesses, or taken when going to war.   Also, the parings of the root, dried in the sun and mixed with salt, are chewed for similar effects. The action seems to be first excitation, followed by depression according to dose and individual temperament, habituation, etc., and it may be fatal. It is considered to be as harmful as *Cannabis*, and crimes attributed to the latter are often really the result of indulgence in niando, or of both used together.   Dalziel

Alhagi maurorum: Arabian manna

The manna or the sweet exudation found on the leaves and branches, known as taranjabin (in India), is given with milk as a restorative and aphrodisiac.   Dastur

19

Allium cepa: Onion
The continuall use, especially of the seeds thereof, engendreth naturall seed and lust.   Langham, 1633

Their Seed provokes Venery.   Short, 1746

A. porrum: Leeks
Nature to restore, stampe Leeke heads very small, and seethe them in water with marrowbones, and the flesh withall.   Then breake them a little, and boyle them a little more, then take out the marrow, and put it into the pot againe with worts [healing herbs] that have been boyled, then strein it, and put thereto powder of pepper, ginger, cinamom, and nutmegs, and eate thereof first and last.   Langham

Leeks provoke the Menses and Spitting, stimulate the Seed Vessels, and excite Venery.   Short

A. sativum: Garlic
Garlic is us'd by Country People to promote the menstrual Flux, and to play unwarrantable Pranks with, of this Kind.   Infus'd in Rhenish [white wine], it provokes powerfully. 'Tis pity so useful a Thing should be so offensive.
The Family Companion for Health, 1730

There is one spice or condiment of which I hesitate to speak, because it is held in such contempt and disdain in this country [England]. I refer to garlic. There can, however, be no question as to its *pronounced aphrodisiac effect.* In fact it stands at the very head of the list. But many of our Anglo-Saxons would perhaps prefer their impotence to the alternative of having to eat garlic. The nations, however, who have no such loathing against the bulb of *allium sativum,* the Italians and Jews for instance, often make

20

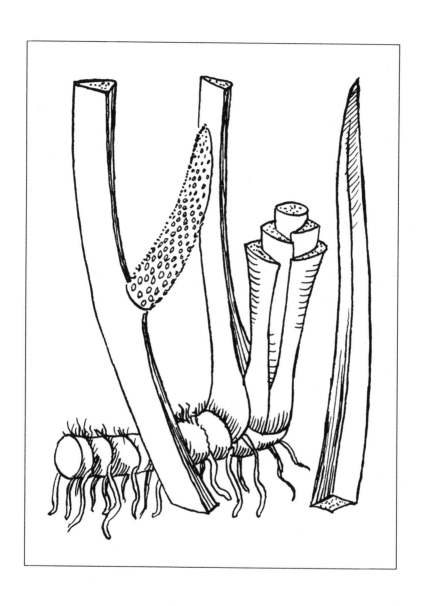

CALAMUS
(Acorus calamus)
See page 18

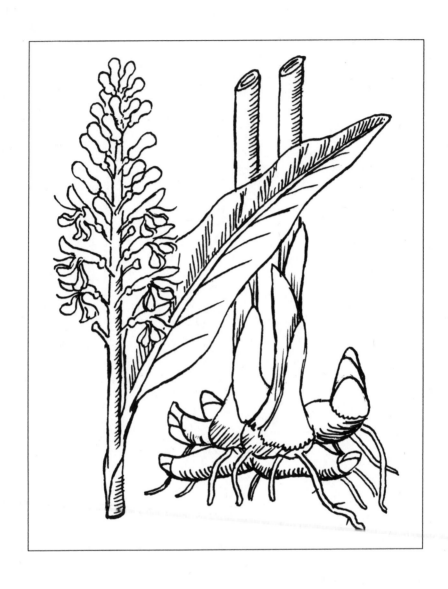

GALANGAL
(*Alpina galanga*)
See page 21

use of garlic as an aphrodisiac; some do it without deliberations, instinctively, so to say. I was told by two or three patients that a druggist was selling an ointment which was very good for impotence. As I am not in the habit of sneering at anything without investigation, and as I always like to consider suggestions no matter from what source they may come, I investigated the matter and found that it was an ointment made from crushed and strained garlic and lard. A small quantity of this was rubbed into the penis and on the back. While the result is, of course, temporary, it is undoubtedly beneficial.   Robinson

Alpinia galanga: Galangal or galanga

The rhizome is a carminative and stomachic, with a reputation among the Arabs as an aphrodisiac.   Burkill

Galangal was formerly much used in Europe as a spice. The root is aromatic, spicy and pungent, resembling a mixture of pepper and ginger. Now used mainly in sauces, curries, liqueurs and bitters.

Amaranthus polygamus: Prince's feathers

The leaves, roots and seeds are used medicinally. A decoction, one in ten, of the leaves and roots is given in one to two ounce doses for impotence.   Dastur

Amaranthus spinosus: Spiny pigweed

The seeds are considered to have the property of brightening the intellect, assisting in the excretory processes, and benefiting the virile powers. Some varieties of this plant are much cultivated and eaten as pot-herbs in China.   Stuart

It is recorded as a cattle and pig food in Indo-China, and as regards cows, is claimed to increase the milk. It is given to cattle in India boiled with pulse to increase the yield of milk.   Burkill

21

Ambergris

Ambergris is a morbid secretion from the sperm whale. Lumps of the waxy formation are found floating on the seas or cast upon beaches. Because of its scarcity, the genuine article is very valuable and often adulterated. Ambergris is used mainly in fine perfumes to fix odors and to impart a rich soft fragrance. Boswell wrote three grains of ambergris taken internally would suffice to produce a marked acceleration of the pulse, a considerable development of muscular strength, a greater activity in the intellectual faculties, and a disposition to cheerfulness and venereal desires. The same author also says that it is a medicine which can, for a short time, restore an effete old man to juvenility. The ancients reposed great confidence in the virtues of this drug, employing it as a renovator of the vital powers and of the organs, whose energy had been exhausted by age or by excess; and throughout the East this perfume still maintains a reputation for life preserving qualities.   Davenport, 1869

American ginseng (See **Panax quinquefolia**)

Anacardium occidentale: Cashew

The fruit of anacardium is well known to West Indians, who, besides eating it in the fresh state, make conserves of it in various ways. Though sweet, it is at the same time very astringent and said to be useful in cases of dysentery and diarrhea. Many and various are the effects with which this tree, its fruit, bark, leaves, and seeds are credited; and if all were true, it would indeed be one of the wonders of nature. It is said to possess aphrodisiacal properties, the leaves to be capable of producing drunkenness, the nuts or seed when roasted to excite the faculties, especially memory, so much so that a confection made therefrom has been called "confection des sages."   Cook and Collins

(See **Semcarpus anacardium** for Oriental variety of cashew. Also called **marking nut**.)

22

Anethum graveolens: Dill

Common oyle, in which Dill is boyled or sunned, as we do oyle of Roses, doth digest, mitigate paine, procureth sleepe, bringeth raw and unconcocted humors to perfect digestion, and proveketh bodily lust.   Gerarde, 1636

Dill seed and herb were often used with other "magic" herbs and seeds in exotic love philters and aphrodisiacs. (See **Anethum** in **Anaphrodisiacs.**)

Anise. (See **Pimpinella anisum**)

Anthriscus cerefolium: Chervil

It is good for people that be dull, old, and without courage, for it rejoiceth and comforteth them, and increaseth their strength.
                                                             Dodoens, 1586

It hath in it a certain windinesse, by means whereof it procureth lust.   Gerarde, 1636

Chervill may be used in pottage, broths, and sallads, etc. In sallads with other herbs it is most acceptable, by reason that it giveth unto them a very pleasant and delicate relish; but for sallads, the seeds while they are green, or the round tufts or heads which containe the seed, do far excell the leaves, which for pleasantness of taste, sweetnesse of smell, and wholsomenesse for every age and temperature, do also excell all other sallad hearbs. And to be eaten by themselves as a sallad, with Oyle, Omphacine, Vinegar, and Pepper, they exceed any other sallad for a cold and feeble stomack. The roots of Chervill boiled, and after dressed, as the cunning cook best knoweth, or only eaten in manner of a sallad with Oyle and Vinegar, are singularly good and wholsome for weak and aged people, and for such as are dull and without courage; for they delight the stomack, rejoice and confort the heart, encrease strength, excite Venus, and depell old age.   Venner, 1650

23

Chervil is much of the Nature of Parsly, being aperitive and attenuating, good for the Stone and Gravel, and to provoke Urine and the Menses. It is more used as a Sallad-Herb then for any Physical use.   J. Miller, 1722

Chervil eaten both boiled and raw in Salads with other Herbs; being a little pleasant it disposes to Venery.   Short, 1746

Apium graveolens: Celery
Potter's *Cyclopaedia* attributes aphrodisiac properties to the seed and *Les Plantes et Les Legumes D'Haiti* attributes aphrodisiac virtue to the root. The following recipe is from the Haitian source: In 1 litre of scalding hot water steep 3 pieces of celery root. Allow to macerate 1/2 hour; sweeten with sugar. Drink wineglassful every 1/4 hour.

The celery root mentioned in the above recipe most likely refers to the wild plant, not to the Apium graveolens var. dulce, the species developed for its succulent stalks. The medicinal properties of garden celery probably is much modified or lost. Guilfoyle stated that the cultivation of celery has removed certain toxic qualities peculiar to the plant in the wild state.

Arctium lappa: Burdock
The stalke of Burdock before the burres come forth, the rinde [skin] pilled off, being eaten raw with salt and pepper, or boyled in the broth of fat meate, is pleasant to be eaten; being taken in that manner it increaseth seed and stirreth lust.
                                        Parkinson, 1629

Laurembergius says that peeled Burdock Stalks, either eaten raw, or boiled very soft, dress'd and eaten, excite Venery much.
                                        Short, 1746

24

Millspaugh wrote (1887), "The herb is so rank that man, the jackass, and caterpiller are the only animals that will eat it." The burs of burdock have distributed this foreign plant over much of America.

Artemisia abrotanum: Southernwood, old man, lad's love, boy's love
If but a branch be laid under the bed's head, they say it provoketh venerie.   Gerarde, 1636

Southernwood was grown in every cottage garden for its aromatic fragrance and dense gray foliage. The slightest contact with the plant fills the air with its lemon-like scent. The dried herb makes an agreeable herb tea if not steeped too long. The plant was formerly in great repute as a cordial against hysterics and to strengthen the stomach of a weak person.

A. absinthium: Wormwood
Absinthe is a liqueur concocted from wormwood and is said to have powerful aphrodisiac properties when not overindulged. The oil of wormwood and the habitual use of absinthe liqueur are narcotic poisons. The herb used as a tea is very popular in Europe in domestic practice for debility and enfeebled digestion. It is considered a tonic, stomachic, febrifuge and anthelmintic. The weak infusion, either made with hot water or the herb steeped in cold water is not toxic if not habitually used and made only with the flowering tops of the herb.

Artichokes. (See Cynara scolymus)

Artocarpus heter-phyllus: jak fruit tree
Tavera says that, according to Father Mercado, the roasted seeds have an aphrodisiac action.   Quisumbing

25

The jak fruit is one of the largest borne by any tree; it ranges in weight from twenty to thirty pounds, but in tropical Asia some varieties produce fruits attaining a weight of seventy to eighty pounds. The soft whitish pulp contains numerous large, nut-like seeds which constitute a valuable part of the fruit. The roasted seeds are a valuable food, and are much relished throughout the tropics.   Sturrock

Ash tree. (See **Fraxinus excelsior**)

Asparagus officinalis: Asparagus
The roots are thought to increase seed and stir up lust.
                                                                Gerarde, 1636

The infusion of asparagus roots drank every Morning several Days together excites Venereal Desire.   Short, 1746

As a food, asparagus is rich. Like germinating peas and beans, it contains an abundance of aminosuccinamic acid, or asparagine, so called as it was isolated first from asparagus.   Burkill

Aspilia latifolia: Haemorrhage plant
Amongst the Hausas the superstitious uses are prominent, as a love philtre, etc.; a charm prepared from the plant and tied around the forehead attracts the "glad eye"; or a youth hides the plant in a maiden's house.
In Liberia it is said the plant is preferred as a haemostatic to any European remedy and to be extraordinarily effective in stopping bleeding, even from a severed artery, as well as inducing rapid healing of the wound. The fresh plant is always used.   Dalziel

Avena satina: Oats
It is a most useful remedy in all cases of nervous exhaustion, general debility, nervous palpitation of the heart, insomnia, inability

26

to keep the mind fixed upon any one subject, etc.; more especially when any or all of these troubles is apparently due to nocturnal emissions, masturbation, over-sexual intercourse, and the like. For these disorders it is truly specific.

Preparation: The fresh green plant, gathered in August, is pounded to a pulp and macerated with 2 parts by weight of alcohol. The usual dose is 15 drops 3 or 4 times a day diluted in water. Anshutz, source of above information, also believed oats "is one of the most valuable means for overcoming the bad effects of the morphine habit."

Averroa carambola: Carmbola
Sanyal and Ghose report that the drug acts as a stimulant to the reproductive organs in both the male and the female. In the female it also increases the fluid of milk and the menstrual fluid. In large doses it acts as an emmengogue like ergot and produces abortion. It is generally administered in the form of an infusion or decoction of the crushed seeds, though it may also be given in the form of a tincture. Like *Cannabis indica*, it has slight intoxicating properties. Quisumbing

Avicennia species: Mangrove
A green bitter and somewhat aromatic resin oozes from the bark. This resin is considered medicinal about the Indian Ocean. An Arab writer calls it an aphrodisiac, and adds that it may also be applied for toothache. Burkill

Balanophora species
A small genus of parasitic leafless herbs, found from India to the New Hebrides. They draw their nourishment from the underground parts of various woody plants, making a knot of stem-tissue in contact with them, perhaps of the size of a fist, from which arises a short, upright, usually coral-red inflorescence. This upright inflorescence is possibly inactive physiologically; but it is

used as an aphrodisiac, its phalloid appearance suggesting the use. (Ridley in *Journ. Straits Med. Assoc.* 5, 1897, p. 123).   Burkill

Barrenwort. (See **Epimedium sagittatum**)

Bauhinia tomentosa

The seeds may be eaten for their tonic and aphrodisiac action.

Nadkarni

Bauhinia pods (especially *B. esculenta*) are an important source of food in Africa where the tree is found. Varieties of Bauhinia *(B. variegata, B. purpurea, B. alba)* are widely planted in Florida for their showy flowers. Commonly known as orchid tree.

Bixa orellana: Anatto, arnatto, lipstick plant

Anatto is much used in domestic medicine in tropical America and aphrodisiac properties have been ascribed to it. The pulp, if applied immediately to burns, is said to prevent the formation of blisters or scars. The leaves are applied as poultices to relieve headache. A decoction of them is employed as a gargle for sore throat. The seeds are said to be the best antidote for poisoning by the manihot plant.

Heckel's *Les Plantes Utiles de Madagascar,* 1910, states that in Madagascar, where the plant is cultivated, the Malagaches who have to speak or dance in public take an infusion of the leaves to make themselves bold and courageous. In Brazil the pulp of the seeds has been given to bulls about to appear in the ring in order to make them more lively and dangerous. It may be that the plant contains some excitant principle which has not yet been investigated.

Bombax malabaricum or B. heptaphylla: Silk-cotton tree

The fruits are used in India for weakness of the genital organs and in most of the disorders in which gentian and calumba are resorted to.   Nadkarni

Gentian and calumba are often used in tonics. The bark of the stem is mucilaginous; its infusion is given as a demulcent and aphrodisiac in seminal weakness.   Dastur

Borreria hispida: Shaggy button weed

Dymock, Warden, and Hooper state that in the Konkan the plant is eaten with other herbs as a vegetable. It is used as a tonic and stimulant in Martinique.

According to Drury and Dymock the roots possess properties similar to those of sarsaparilla. They are prescribed in decoction as a alterative.

Dymock, Warden, and Hooper state the seeds are thought to be aphrodisiac.   Quisumbing

Brassica alba or nigra: Mustard

An Electuary of the seeds excites Venery.   Short, 1746

Davenport mentions several cases were cured of atony of the virile member of three or four years' duration, by repeated immersions of that organ in a strong infusion of mustard seed.

B. rapa: Turnip

They are a good Pectoral, Diuretic, and increase Seed; half a Dram of the seed, drank, excites Venery.   Short

In 1934 a researcher of the University of Toronto School of Hygiene reported the juice from the lowly turnip (roots) was a good substitute for orange or tomato juice as a natural source of vitamin C. The juice is said to be sweet and not unpalatable.

29

Brillantaisia patula

The plant is a familiar medicine, sometimes grown in native gardens in Lagos, used by a bride or a barren wife to ensure conception.   Dalziel

Burdock. (See Arctium lappa)

Calamus. (See Acorus calamus)

Cannabis sativa: Marijuana

All parts of the plant (especially the female plant) are narcotic. In moderate doses the plant is at first an exhilarant and powerful aphrodisiac; after a while it is sedative.   Its habit leads to indigestion, body-waste, melancholia and impotence.   In large doses it first produces mental exaltation, intoxication, a sense of double consciousness and finally loss of memory, gloominess, etc.   Nadkarni

Since Nadkarni's statement was made the use of marijuana has become world-wide, and unsuspecting human guinea pigs are beginning to reveal more effects from its use. Evidence now indicates when marijuana is smoked during pregnancy there is a much higher incidence of malformed babies. There is evidence that heavy use of marijuana may lead to temporary sterility. In preadolescent males an imbalance in testosterone may adversely affect puberty and normal maturation. Researchers also believe there is greater vulnerability to diseases among marijuana users.

Marijuana is also known as hemp, and the strong fiberous stems of the plant are used in the manufacture of cordage, hangman's rope and coarse textile fabrics. The seed was once used for cage birds and is said to greatly increase the brilliancy of their plumage, and, in the case of the bullfinch and some others, to cause it to turn black. Hemp seeds also yield a useful oil.

Cantharis vesicatoria: Spanish fly, blister beetle

Of all aphrodisiacs, the most certain and terrible in its effects are cantharides, commonly known as Spanish fly. That they exercise a powerful and energetic action upon the organization and stimulate, to the utmost, the venereal desire, is but too true. The effects, however, which these insects, when applied as a blister upon the skin, are known to produce, are insignificant when compared with their intense action upon the stomach when taken internally; nor is it the stomach only which is affected by them: the bladder experiences an irritation exceeding even that caused by the severest strangury. To these succeed perforation of the stomach, ulcers, throughout the entire length of the intestinal canal, dysentery, and, lastly, death in the midst of intolerable agonies.

Davenport, 1869

In India another insect was used like Spanish fly and apparently also with accompanying dangers. Dey wrote, "This fly, if procured before the mites have commenced its destruction, yields, on the average, one-third more cantharidin than the Spanish fly of the European shops."

Florida also has a species of blister beetle.

Cardamon. (See Elettaria cardamomum)

Carissa edulis: Carissa

The root is regarded as a tonic, to restore virility, and was at one time used as bitters, macerated in rum, gin, etc.   Dalziel

Carissa is an attractive evergreen much used as a hedge or fence in Florida. The delicious fruits are dark purple when ripe. The fruits are eaten fresh, in salads, and as a sauce. The flavor is vaguely suggestive of the raspberry.

Carpolobia alba and C. lutea

An African tree that bears sweet edible fruits. In South Nigeria the root is regarded as an invigorating tonic or aphrodisiac, and is an ingredient with the fruit and other medicines in concoctions for sustaining vitality. A similar action of the roots, chewed as a stimulant, is recorded in Cameroons. Dalziel

Carrot. (See Daucus carota)

Cashew. (See Anacardium occidentale)

Catha edulis: Abyssinian tea, khat, gat, quaat, quat

Long before coffee was introduced, aboriginals were chewing the bitter leaves of this shrub as a stimulant and aphrodisiac. Khat is also prepared as tea. Its use is spreading throughout parts of northeastern Africa. It is now banned by Saudi Arabia, Egypt, Somalia, Kenya, and other governments with little effect. It is said Mau Mau tribesmen chew khat for courage to battle encroaching white settlers. In remote areas of the interior of Ethiopia khat leaves are distributed to road workers in order to get a job done. A report states: "After time out for chewing, the picks and shovels fly and the work is speedily completed."

Scientists report khat contains a substance called norpseudo-phedrine and a related constituent, both of which are similar to alkaloids, of amphetamine. The combination stimulates the chewer of khat to vigorous physical activity as adrenalin is released through the body. Analysis also shows khat is rich in vitamin C and contains fair amounts of elements generally found in most leaves.

Like all habit-forming drugs, khat is suspected of having very harmful reactions when habitually and excessively used.

Celery. (See Apium graveolen)

Celosia argentea: Cockscomb
In the Phillippines Guerrero reports that the seeds, when in decoction, or finely powdered, are considered aphrodisiac.

Quisumbing

Cockscomb is a common weed in China and is believed to be the forerunner of the showy plants extensively cultivated in gardens over the world. The wild species is mentioned in old Chinese herbals.

Cetraria islandica: Iceland moss
A 1972 German herbal states Iceland moss is used for symptoms of chronic emaciation, phlegm in fine branches of the windpipe, for weaknesses of muscles and vascular system; for those inclined to consumption; for body weaknesses caused by sexual excesses and to strengthen the lungs. Iceland moss is used as a tonic, rather than an aphrodisiac.

Chamomile. (See Matricaria chamomilla)

Charms, Amulets, Images, etc.
The last battering engines, says Burton, author of *Anatomy of Melancholy*, are philters, amulets, charms, images, and such unlawful meanes: If they cannot prevail of themselves by the help of bawds, panders, and their adherents, they will fly for succor to the devil himself. I know there be those that deny the devil can do any such thing, and that there is no other fascination than that which comes by the eyes. It was given out of old, that a Thessalian wench had bewitched King Philip to dote on her, and by philters enforced his love, but when Olympia, his queen, saw the maid of an excellent beauty well brought up and qualified: these, quoth she, were the philters which enveagled King Philip, these the true charms as Henry to Rosamond.

"One accent from thy lips the blood more warmes
Than all their philters, exorcismes, and charmes."

33

With this alone Lucretia brags, in Aretine, she could do more than all philosophers, astrologers, alchymists, necromancers, witches, and the rest of the crew. As for herbs and philters I could never skill of them. The sole philter I ever used was kissing and embracing, by which alone I made men rave like beasts, stupefied and compelled them to worship me like an idol. Davenport, 1869

Chasmanthera owariensis: Velvet leaf or False Pareira Brava

The root is used as a medicine to prevent a threatened abortion. It is also a secret remedy of African Women to retain conjugal affection.   Dalziel

Chervil. (See Anthriscus cerefolium)

Chicken eggs

W.J. Robinson, noted authority on sexual impotence, said he often made his patients eat two to six raw eggs a day, two or three the first thing in the morning, before breakfast, the rest during the day. He believed it is best to drink the egg directly from the shell making a hold at the top, put in a pinch of salt and sip it.

Egg-nogs were very popular in folk practice for convalescence, for the aged, and to increase virility.

An old fashioned recipe:

Take 2 eggs, 2 tablespoons of powdered sugar, 1/2 pint of milk, 1/2 pint of sweet cream, 6 tablespoons of brandy or whisky. Beat the yolks of the eggs and sugar together until very light. Stir in the milk and cream, and when well-blended with the egg, add brandy or whisky. Lastly, whip in the whites of the eggs, which have been beaten to a stiff froth.

Hot egg-nog:

Take yolk of 1 egg, 1 scant tablespoon of sugar, 1 pint of boiling milk, 2 tablespoons of brandy or whisky. Beat egg and sugar together until quite light, and stir it briskly into the boiling milk. Add brandy or whisky and serve with a little grated nutmeg on top.

Pousse L'Amour: Recipe from *Fancy Drinks and Popular Beverages* (1891).   Fill a sherry glass with the following: 1/3 maraschino; the yolk of 1 fresh egg; 1/3 of creme de roses; 1/3 of brandy.   Raw eggs also may be taken with beer with a dash of pepper.

Chick embryo

Daily doses of one 7 to 9 day-old chick embryo is prescribed by some modern "reconditioning or rejuvenating centers."   They generally cater to professional people who try to keep an ageless appearance before the public.   The live embryo is part of a diet taken for two or three weeks.   It is said (by promoters) the results show marked restoration of vital powers to perform *all* body functions.

Chinese aphrodisiac pill recipe:

Combine *Cyperus rotundus, Pachyma cocos* (the kind that encircles the root), and honey.   For impotence in middle age, and to prolong virility into old age (51-80).   Another formula is as follows: *Atractylis sinensis, Zanthoxylum,* fennel, and paste (probably made from rice).   Tonic and strengthening to the virile powers, producing fertility.   Stuart

Chinese ginseng. (See **Panax ginseng**)

Chocolate. (See **Theobroma cacao**)

Chrysactina mexicana: False damiana

This is a heath-like shrub found in Mexico and Central America, popular among natives who believe it capable of rejuvenating males.   Some years ago in the Institute Medico Nacional, a strong decoction made of branches and leaves was given to several anemia patients and anemia convalescents.   After several weeks of daily doses it was found the decoction, as well as the extract, had no tonic effects as commonly claimed by natives. Natives still believe and use the decoction.

Chrysanthemum sinense: Chrysanthemum
The use of the dew gathered from the flowers is held in much repute in preserving and restoring the vital functions. As to the wild variety, the whole plant is recommended to be used, though it is thought to be slightly poisonous.   Quisumbing

H.L. Li, author of *The Garden Flowers of China* (1959), mentions a popular summer drink known as Chrysanthemum Dew was made by brewing the petals of the flower, then diluting the strained liquid with water.

Cicer arietinum: Chick peas
Spanish Chick Peas are best for Coffee (roasted like coffee), and come nearest it. Chicks contain much Oil and Salt; some eat them freely for Food, but they are a little flatulent, stir up Lust, and some imagine they increase Seed.   Short, M.D., 1746

Cinnamomum parthenoxylon
The bark of this species of cinnamon is considered an excellent tonic, particularly for girls attaining maturity in Malaysian Islands.   Burkill

Clary sage. (See Salvia sclarea)

Claviceps purpurea: Ergot
Ergot has a specific effect on the reproductive organs of both sexes. In parts of Europe ergot sometimes gets into rye-bread (spurred type). Dr. Deslandes, in speaking of the people living in Gironde Valley [France] said, "They present a striking example how violent passions can be associated with weakened frames." Their food is scanty and lacking in nourishing properties, largely composed of rye meal from which the diseased grains have not

36

been separated. Their faces are disfigured, pinched, and pale, and their leanness almost shocking. They present an appearance of complete physical degradation and yet their passions are precocious, and they yield them with real frenzy. Napheys, 1871

Ergot is a dangerous poison for those not familiar with its use.

Cnicus japonicus or Carduus acaulis
The root, which has a sweetish pleasant taste, is the part used in medicine. Very remarkable virtues are ascribed to it, such as building up the animal spirits and restoring the blood.   Stuart

Uphof states the young leaves are eaten as a vegetable in Japan.

Cocaine. (See Erythroxylon coca)

Cocculus cordifolius: Heart-leaved moonseed
The entire plant is regarded (in India) as a valuable alterative and tonic.

Besides being a tonic and rejuvenator, it is indicated in several diseases attended with great debility.   Nadkarni

Heart-leaved moonseed is a common climbing shrub found in tropical Western India.

Coriandrum sativum: Coriander
The seed was a popular ingredient of love potions during the Middle Ages, probably only to add flavor. The seed is said to contain large amounts of vitamin A.

Costus speciosus
The powdered herb taken internally is considered to be tonic, depurative and aphrodisiac in the Malayan Islands. The plant is also used in occult and magic practice.   Burkill

37

Cotton. (See **Gossypium herbaceum**)

Cowhage or cowitch. (See **Mucuna pruriens**)

Cress. (See **Lepidium sativum**)

Crocus sativus: Saffron
Sodden in wine and drunke, it preserveth from drunkennesse,
and provoketh lust.   Langham, 1633

It provoketh urine, stirreth fleshly lust.   Gerarde, 1636

Flowers taken in a moderate Dose quicken the Senses, shake off
Dullness, but too much cause Watchings, Sleepiness or Pain of the
Head. . . . All Agree that Saffron is a great Cordial, and causes
Chearfulness;. . .excites Venery.   Short, 1746

In small doses it acts as a mild stimulant, and in large doses as
an aphrodisiac.   Dastur

Col. Sir R. N. Chopra wrote: "As a stimulant and aphrodisiac,
it is considered to be a sovereign remedy, not to be excelled in
virtue by the whole range of drugs in the Materia Medica."
                                                           Nadkarni

Cubebs. (See **Piper cubeba**)

Curculigo orchioides:
The root, when powdered and used pure, or mixed with other
tonic or carminative vegetable drugs, is considered tonic, pectoral,
diuretic and aphrodisiac.
Kirtikar and Basu, Nadkarni, Drury, and Dey report that the root
is aromatic and slightly bitter, and mucilagenous to the taste, and
is considered demulcent, diuretic and restorative.   Quisumbing

Cuscuta species: Dodder

Aphrodisiac properties were ascribed to the seeds of this wiry parasite by the Chinese. It was believed if taken for a long time, they would brighten the eye, enliven the body, and prolong life.

Stuart

An African dodder is used as a charm. When a young man wants to know the availability of a particular female, he hangs some dodder on a tree. If the plant does not grow he assumes he would be rejected. The youth probably would have better luck if he placed the plant on a tree which dodder grows best on.

Cycas circinalis: Ceylon sago

The male bracts are used as narcotic; they have a property that intoxicates insects that rest upon them; also stimulant and aphrodisiac.

Bracts or scales contain in a dried state much albuminous and mucilaginous matter soluble in water; but no alkaloid or other principles found that would account for its narcotic actions, but a glucoside "pakocin" is found. It yields a gum resembling tragacanth and also a kind of sago or flour.   Nadkarni

Cyclamen europaeum: Sowbread, ground bread

It is used for women in long and hard travels where there is danger, to accelerate the birth, either the roote or the leafe being applyed. But for any amorous effects, I hold it meere fabulous.

Parkinson, 1629

Cyclamen is the attractive house plant offered in many florist shops. Nickell lists the root as acrid, bitter, drastic poison and, of course, should not be used internally.

Cymbopogon schoenanthus: Camel grass

The internal part of the rhizome is said to be eaten as an aphrodisiac.   Dalziel

39

Uphof mentions the grass is a source of essential oil used for medicinal purposes and sometimes in perfumes. It was esteemed in early civilizations.

Cynara scolymus: Artichokes

Being boyled, and eaten with butter, pepper, and a little vinegar, they are accounted a dainty dish, and restorative, being very pleasant to the taste, acceptable to the stomack, and powerful for exciting of Venus, and therefore an excellent nourishment for them that are weak in their genitall parts.   Venner, 1650

Gerarde (1636) believed artichokes only stirred up gas. He wrote: In my judgement, which way soever they be drest and eaten, they stirre and cause a filthy loathsom stinking winde within the body, thereby causing the belly to be pained and tormented; and are a meat more fit for swine.

Salmon (1710) gives this manner of preparing the thistle-like heads: Take an artichoke, and dress it with milk; that is, first boil your artichokes in water till the leaves will just draw off; put them in new milk; and boil them thoroughly; bruise the pulp in the milk, and add a little mace and grated nutmeg, sweeten it with sugar, and eat often of it with a spoon. It exceedingly restores decayed vigour, and strengthens not only the spirits, but the whole frame of the body. The Germans and French usually eat the tender stalks of this plant boiled with butter and vinegar; the Italians seldom boil the heads, but eat them raw, with salt, pepper, oil and vinegar; they are moreover held to provoke venery, and the decoction of the buds drank provoke urine.

Jacques Kother, author of *Memoirs of a Belly,* states the French were already very fond of artichokes four hundred years ago, to which they attributed aphrodisiac qualities. Catherine de Medici used to make meals consisting of nothing but artichokes and cock's kidneys.

40

Cyperus esculentus: Earth nut, earth almond.

Either raw, or boiled in Broth, eaten with Butter and Pepper after they are peeled, are pleasant, common, nourishing Food, and provoke Venery according to Lauremberguis.   Short, 1746

The earth nut is widely regarded as having an aphrodisiac affect.   Dalziel

Earth nut has been cultivated since early times. The tuberous rootstocks are used as food for man and hogs. A beverage is made of the juice of pressed tubers.

Damiana: (See Turnera diffusa var. aphrodisiaca)

Datura species

Varieties of this plant are found over much of the tropics as well as far into the northern and southern hemispheres of the world. Because of *Datura's* wide distribution, it has been since ancient times proved the most dangerous of all plants to Homo sapien species. Death was caused by ignorance, mere inquisitiveness, foolhardy daring or evil intention.

The seeds of *D. stramonium* have the effect of producing delirium, and are said to have been used by the priests of Apollo at Delphi to produce their ravings, which were called prophecies. In Haiti *D. stramonium* is known as "concombre zombi" or "zombi cucumber." Peasants use branches of the fresh plant to put under the pillow in order to "make one sleep."

Datura arborea and *D. sanguinea* are large bushed natives of Peru often planted in tropical countries for their attractive hanging flowers. The seeds of these varieties are also narcotic. South American Indians make a drink of *A. arborea and A. sanguinea,* believing the brew could bring them into communication with spirits of their forefathers. Most likely some Indians joined their forefathers soon after partaking of the deadly decoction.

41

East Indian botanist Dastur reported all parts of *Datura* metal are strongly intoxicant, narcotic, aphrodisiac and tonic. Nadkarni claimed the black variety (*D. fastuosa*) of Asiatic origin is more potent and aphrodisiac. *Datura* species were used by East Indian poisoners who gave them not with the intention of killing, but of stupefying their victims for the purpose of facilitating theft and expediting other evil designs.

Daucus carota: Carrot

The root boiled and eaten, or boiled in wine, and the decoction drunk provoketh urine, expelleth the stone, bringeth forth the birth; it also procureth bodily lust. 　　　　　　　　　　Gerarde, 1636

The wild carrot or Queen Anne's Lace is the original of the cultivated carrot. All parts of the wild species is used in folk practice for affections of the bladder. (See *American Folk Medicine* by Clarence Meyer.)

Dendrobium macrael: Indian orchid

The plant, root and stems are used in India as a tonic for debility due to seminal discharges. The whole plant is used in decoction along with other drugs having similar properties.

　　　　　　　　　　　　　　　　　　　　Nadkarni

Dendrobium is one of the most popular of all orchids and also one of the largest genus. Some six hundred species range from India and Ceylon to Australia, New Zealand, Japan, and Pacific Islands. There are also many artificially produced hybrids.

Dill. (See Anethum graveolens)

Dodder. (See Cuscuta)

Dracaena graminifolia

Hooper reports that the candied tubers are eaten as a medicine and are regarded as tonic and aphrodisiac.

Durio zibethinus: Durian

Much has been written about this large spiny fruit of the *Durio* trees found in the wilds of Indonesia, Sumatra, the Celebes, the Moluccas, and Borneo. Naturalists and botanists agree on two points: the fruit stinks, and the flavor of the pulp is out of this world. The odor and flavor descriptions of the durian are as different as the nose and taste buds of each writer. One author believed the odor resembled gorganzola cheese; another described it as a mixture of old cheese and onions flavored with turpentine; a highly sensitive writer compared durian with French custard that was dragged through a sewer pipe. The odor and flavor of the fruit also attracts elephants, tigers and other wild animals and, needless to say, every insect in the jungle. As the fruit decays rapidly, natives camp around the durian tree in order to be on hand when they ripen.

The Malaysians have long regarded durian fruit as highly nutritious, as well as being an aphrodisiac. It apparently was the *elixir vitae* for one of Indonesia's highest officials who had a reputation for his devotion to the fair sex. The official was photographed eating durian while attending the cornerstone-laying ceremony at the new University of Indonesia in 1965.

According to Ochse, an aromatic herb (*Limnophilia*) is eaten raw or steamed and thought to be good for quieting the stomach after durians are eaten.

Echinops echinatus: Globe-Thistle

All parts of the plant are used. It forms a chief ingredient in various alterative, tonic decoctions for impotence and seminal debility.
Nadkarni

Several varieties of globe-thistle are found in Europe. *Echinops ritro* is grown in gardens for its unique ball-like blue flowers.

Egg plant. (See **Solanum melongena**)

Eggs. (See **Chicken eggs**)

Elettaria cardamomum: Cardamon

The exotic fragrance of this pod appears to be particularly seductive to Arabs as it is considered to have had great powers as an aphrodisiac with them since ancient times. Cardamons were often used in love potions. In the Western World the pods are much used in Christmas cookies, Danish and Swedish coffee cakes, pastries and candies. In the Orient the pods are used in curries and assorted dishes. Persians steep a pod in their coffee after it has brewed, and the French use it in their demi-tasse. The pods are chewed as a breath-sweetener, especially to cover up bad taste and tell-tale alcohol breath. They are also much used as an ingredient in potpourri and sachet mixtures.

Epimedium sagittatum: Barrenwort

This plant is common in the mountain valleys throughout China. Goats eating the plant are said to be incited to excessive copulations, hence the Chinese name Yin-yang-hus. The root and leaves are prescribed in sterility and barrenness, and is said to have great virtues in these conditions.   Stuart

They [leaves] have the reputation of being a powerful aphrodisiac and useful in kidney troubles.   *Gardens Bulletin*

Ergot. (See **Claviceps purpurea**)

Eruca sativa: Garden rocket

The plant Rocket has been especially celebrated by the ancient poets for possessing the virtue of restoring vigor to the sexual

44

organs, on which account it was consecrated to and sown around, the statue of Priapus.

Thus Columella says:

> Th' eruca, Priapus, near thee we sow.
> To rouse to duty husbands who are slow.

Virgil attributes to it the same quality:

> Th' eruca plant which gives to jaded appetite the spur.

Lobel gives an amusing account of the effects of this plant upon certain monks in the garden of whose monastery it was sown, an infusion of it being daily doled out to them under the impression that its cheering and exhilarating qualities would rouse them from the state of inactivity and sluggishness so common to the inmates of such establishments. But, alas! the continual use of it produced an effect far more powerful than had been contemplated by the worthy itinerant monk who had recommended it, for the poor cenobites were so stimulated by its aphrodisiacal virtues that, transgressing alike their monastic walls and vows, they sought relief for their amorous desires in the fond embraces of the women residing in the neighborhood.   Davenport, 1869

The use therof [rocket] stirreth up bodily pleasure, especially of the seed, also it provoketh urine, and helpeth the digestion of the meates.   Dodoens, 1586

Rockets gives Salads a fine Taste, and the same it does to Sauces and Seasonings; it is grateful to the Palate, excites Lust, and is said to increase Seed.   Short, 1746

Aphrodisiac properties were still ascribed to rocket in Whitlaw's *New Medical Discoveries*, 1829.

Eryngium species

Pliny the Elder wrote the following almost 2,000 years ago: The whole variety of the Eryngium known in our (the Latin) language as the *centum capita* has some marvellous facts recorded of it.   It is said to bear a striking likeness to the organs of generation of either sex; it is rarely met with, but if a root resembling the male organ of the human species be found by a man, it will ensure him woman's love; hence it is that Phaon, the Lesbian, was so passionately beloved of Sappho.   If it be true, as is asserted by medical writers, that the above root contains an essential oil of peculiarly stimulating qualities, the fact would account, not only for Sappho's passion for Phaon, but also for the high value set upon it by the rival wives of Jacob.

Eryngium maritimum: Sea Holly
The apothecaries of this countrey doe use to preserve and comfit the roote of Eryngium, to be given to the aged and old people, and others that are consumed or withered, to nourish and restore them agayne.   Dodoens, 1586

Iringo-roots are hot and dry in the second degree, with a tenuity of substance: they strengthen the stomack and liver, discusse wind, and are of an excellent efficacy for all infirmities of the kidneyes, both clensing and strengthening Them.   The roots condited, or preserved with Sugar, do exceedingly refresh and comfort the body, and restore the naturall moisture. They are very greatly availeable for old and aged people, and for such as are weake by nature, refreshing and restoring the one, and amending the defects of nature in the other. They excite and give ability to venereall embracements.   Venner, 1650

The candied Root is thought to be a Stimulus to Venery.
                                                        Short, 1746

E. campestre: Field eryngo
The root is sweet, aromatic and tonic. Boerhaave reckons it as the first of aperient diuretic roots. It has been recommended in gonorrhoea, suppression of the menses, and visceral obstructions,

46

particularly of the gall bladder and liver; it has also the credit of being a decided aphrodisiac. A good deal of candied root is still sold. *E. maritimum* has similar properties but in a less degree.

Lindley, 1838

E. maritimum

The candied roots were sold in shops under the name of kissing comfits. Rhind, 1868

E. coeruleum

The root is used in northwestern India as a tonic and is supposed to be aphrodisiac. Burkill

Eryngium comosum: Yerba del sapo

The juice or a concentrated decoction from the root of this plant is used as a diuretic and aphrodisiac for contractions of the womb. It is also recommended for gonorrhea. Martinez

E. aquaticum: Water eryngo

The author of a very recent publication mentions *Eryngium aquaticum* used for sexual exhaustion and loss of erectile powers. *Eryngium aquaticum* is a native American species and this writer has never found such attributes in early American or ethnobotany records.

Eryngium aquaticum appears to have been more than an aphrodisiac. Anshutz mentions several cases where the botanical cured damaged testicles. In one instance a married man injured his testicles by jumping upon a horse; this was followed by a discharge of what was considered semen for fifteen years, during which time he was treated allopathically and homocopathically. Dr. Parks exhibited a number of the usual remedies without permanent benefit. He then gave a half-grain dose, three times a day, of the third decimal trituration of the *Eryngium aquaticum*. In five days the emissions were entirely suppressed, and had not returned during

47

a period of two years. The emissions were without erections day or night, and were followed by great lassitude.

Erythroxylon coca: Bolivian coca, cocaine (Not to be confused with **cocoa** or **chocolate**.)

The highly stimulating property of coca leaves probably was another discovery of the ancient Incas, and like *Panax Ginseng* it was reserved only for the use of royalty or people of distinction, such as high officials, priests and warriors. After the conquest of the Incas, Spanish taskmasters doled the coca leaves out to Indian slaves and laborers in order to get more work done without increasing their daily diet. Coca leaves have a reputation of making Indians of the Andes invulnerable to the heat of gold mines, the cold of high altitude, and to hunger and thirst. The use of coca became so habitual that the cheeks of many Indians bulge out permanently from the wad of leaves kept in the mouth. The pouchbelt containing coca leaves was as indispensable to the Indian as any article of clothing worn. Coca leaves were chewed with lime made by burning bones, shells, or the leaves of cecropia tree. In a pinch, ash of the campfire is used. It was believed the lime gave the chewer maximum effect of coca leaves with less reaction.

Like many other habit forming drugs, the use of coca leaves and its active constituent is spreading over a world that has become easily accessible by land, water and air.

The following excerpts from East Indian doctors refers to the alkaloid cocaine--the magic local anesthetic, which of course is far more potent than chewing the leaves of the bush:

It [cocaine] is popularly believed to be a sexual stimulant, and it has a most extraordinary effect, temporary though it be, in rapidly overcoming mental as well as physical fatigue. The prolonged abuse brings about gradual development of grave symptoms. Nadkarni

48

In poisonous doses death is due to paralysis of the heart and respiration and is preceded by convulsions. About one gram of cocaine is sufficient to kill an adult unless he is gradually habituated to it, in which case much larger doses are borne, as in the case opium. In chronic cocaine-eaters the most characteristic symptom is the feeling of the presence of sand, worms, or insects (cocaine bugs) under the skin (Magnam's symptom).

Dr. M.A. Kamatt

A 1974 report states that new laboratory findings concerning cocaine reveals that the addicted use of cocaine has a greater potential for abuse than heroin. (See **Erythroxylon** in **Anaphrodisiacs**)

Euadenia eminens

In Africa the peppery seeds are chewed. The pulp around the seeds is said to be an effective aphrodisiac. According to Chevalier the plant is poisonous.

Dalziel

Euchrestia horsfieldii

Burkill reports that the seeds are tonic with an aphrodisiac action; but they are so poisonous that great caution is required in their use.

Eugenia crenulata: Zo douvant

In Haiti, the leaves are referred to as "so-so with a head." Peasants steep the leaves in rum as an aphrodisiac. The leaves are also much used in herb charm mixtures tied up in small bundles of various colored cloths. The bundles known as "voodoo ouanges" or "wangas" are tapered at ends where cloth is brought together then topped with cock feathers. Ogun, the loa of war and fertility, is represented with bright red cloth; Erzulie, goddess of love and most popular of all loas, is represented in light blue cloth.

Eulophia campestris: Witton root
Tubers contain large quantities of white mucilage and ash 3.6 percent. Used as nutritive, tonic, and aphrodisiac. Said to be a fair substitute for salep (*Orchis mascula*).   Nadkarni

Euphorbia convolvuloides
Applied to women's breasts the latex is supposed to increase lactation (probably by sympathetic magic). It is also used as a love charm by youths and maidens.
                                                                    Dalziel

False damiana: (See **Chrysactina mexicana**)

Fennel. (See **Foeniculum vulgare**)

Fenugreek. (See **Trigonella foenum graecum**)

Ficus religiosa: Peepul, Pagoda or sacred fig tree
In India the bark boiled in milk is said to be a good aphrodisiac.
The alluded property most likely is associated with folklore and other legends of this most sacred tree. Vishnu, the second god of the Hindu triad, was believed to have been born under the Cathedral-like (Nehrling's description) branches of a great peepul tree. The sacred legend was mentioned as early as 400 B.C. by Herodotus and later by Pliny and Steabo.

Flax seed. (See **Linum usitatissimum**)

Foeniculum vulgare: Fennel
Seethe the tufts of Fennel in wine, potage, or ale, to helpe the bladder, reines, and stone, and to increase milke and naturall seed. The seed stirreth man to procreation.
                                                            Langham, 1633

50

F. vulgare var. dulce or F. var. azoricum: Finocchio, Florence fennel

The stalk is reported to be eaten in Apulia roasted in embers, first wrapped in leaves or in old clouts, with pepper and salt; which, as they say, is a pleasant sweet food, that stirreth up lust, as they report.   Gerarde, 1636

Fraxinus excelsior: European ash

Ash-keys [seeds], commonly called Kite-keys of the Ash, being while they are young boyled and preserved in pickle made of Vinegar and Salt, make a most wholsom and profitable sauce to excite the appetite, mundifie the stomack, and to open the obstructions of the Spleen and Liver. Moreover they provoke urine, and incite to Venus. This sauce of Ash-keys is very profitable for them that have weak and windy stomacks, especially for the elder sort of people, and such as are subject to the stopping of the Spleen and Liver, which parts it doth not only effectually open, but also greatly corroborate.   Venner, 1650

Gerarde mentioned a different recipe. He wrote: "The seed or Ash keyes provoke urine, increase naturall seed, and stirre up bodily lust, especially being poudered with nutmegs and drunke." He also added this interesting tidbit, "Three or foure leaves of the Ash tree taken in wine each morning from time to time, doe make those lean that are fat, and keep them from feeding that begin to wax fat."

Galega officinalis: Goat's rue

Offered by most mail order specialists and at local institutes for bust development, it is claimed that wonderful results have been obtained in many cases, not only as a bust developer, but as an aphrodisiac for women. The discovery of this drug was due to its extensive use in the central parts of Europe, where it is given to cows to increase the quantity of their milk from thirty to fifty percent.   Covey

51

Galega is often grown as an ornamental, but this author found it difficult to control and, if unattended, it would have taken over the entire garden.

Galium luteum: Lady's bed-straw
The root thereof drunke in wine stirreth bodily lust: and the floures smelled unto worke the same effect.   Gerarde, 1636

The roots provoke Lust, and excite to Venery.   Short, 1746

Garcinia mannii: Mangosteen species
A small tree native of West Tropical Africa. It bears fruit somewhat similar to an orange and the acid pulp is relished by the natives. The roots are steeped in palm wine or gin and taken as an aphrodisiac.   Dalziel

The genus *Garcinia* is imperfectly known, there being well over two hundred species in tropical Asia, Africa and Malaysia. There is a great diversity among the species of *Garcinia* in growth form, in the foliage, in the flowers, and in its fruits, which may vary in shape, quality, and color. The best-known and practically the only species with fruits of commercial value at present is the famous mangosteen of tropical Asia.   Sturrock

Garlic. (See Allium sativum)

Ginger. (See Zingiber officinale)

Ginseng. (See Panax)

Glycyrrhiza glabra: Licorice or sweet root
Ancient Chinese made little distinction between foods and medicines and divided their therapeutics into three classes. Those of the first class consisted of simple foods that were least likely to disturb the normal functions of the body, regardless of age and

52

physical condition, even when the article was taken over lengthy periods. Licorice was considered a first class drug and it stood next to ginseng in importance in Chinese pharmacy, being the great corrective adjunct and harmonizing ingredient in a large number of recipes. Stuart wrote, "Like most celebrated Chinese drugs, licorice was credited with property of rejuvenating those who consumed it for a long time."

Licorice plays an important part in medicine according to Brahmanism, the oldest religion of India. It is one of the principle drugs of the "Susruta," a text said to have been revealed by Brahma himself. The revered record of seven hundred and ninety-eight plant medicines recommended licorice as a general tonic, beautifying agent and elixir of life.

Licorice is also important in the Buddhist religion. The infusion of the root is used for bathing Buddha on the annual celebration of his birth, on the eighth day of the eighth month. The infusion is poured over the statue of the god three times with great pomp while the priests chant mystical incantations and the worshippers pray. The fluid which drips from the statue is collected for its supposed curative properties. Licorice is also an ingredient of love potions in India.

Licorice was known to be used by the ancient Sumerian, Egyptian, Greek and Roman physicians. It was an important medicinal throughout the Middle Ages and into modern times. Some nationalities still regard it as an aphrodisiac. In the Spanish speaking island of the West Indies licorice root is steeped in rum. In Polish communities of some large American cities the root is steeped in whiskey.

Gossypium herbaceum: Cotton

The seede of Cotton swageth the cough, and is good against all cold diseases of the breast, augmenteth naturall strength, and encreaseth the seede of generation.   Dodoens, 1586

It [seed] also stirreth up lust of the body by increasing naturall seed; wherein it surpasseth.   Gerarde, 1636

Cottonseed is an excellent source of vitamin E. A recent report states that cotton flour made from cottonseed contains up to 70 percent protein--more than three times the protein value of beef, pork, poultry or fish, and up to seven times the protein value of wheat flour.

Grains of Paradise. (See **Aframomum melegueta**)

Grammatophyllum speciosum: Letter plant
The seeds of this fantastic orchid are used by natives of Malaysia and Solomon Isles in love philtres.

Letter plant is regarded as the queen of orchids and is the giant and one of the most magnificent of all *epiphytes*. A speciman growing in the Botanical Garden of Buitzenzorg, Java, had the following dimensions: diameter of whole plant, 18 feet; collar about the trunk of the tree formed by closely interwoven roots, 7 1/2 feet; diameter, 2 1/2 feet thick, and over 3 feet high; flower-clusters appearing at the same time, 50 to 60; each 2 feet or more in length. The beautiful deep red-purple spotted yellow flowers are six inches in diameter. Because of its great size the letter plant is little grown in hothouses.

Grewia umbellata
A sprawling shrub found in Siam, Sumatra and Borneo; in the Peninsula it is common in the more occupied parts. The shrub is regarded as aphrodisiac by the natives.   Burkill

There is little available information on the *Grewia*. A variety (*G. denticulata*) that grows in India is described as a small tree resembling a mulberry which bears enormous quantities of acid drupes, about the size of cranberries; used for pickling.

Hibiscus cannabinus: Bimlipitum jute

According to Kirtikar, Basu, and Nadkarni the seeds taken internally are said to be aphrodisiac and fattening. The seeds yield an edible oil.   Quisumbing

The above species was once widely grown in Europe for its fiberous stalks to make cord.

H. esculentus: Okra

In some parts of West Africa mild aphrodisiac properties are attributed to the seeds.   Dalziel

The mucilage (cooked unripe fruit) is considered to have aphrodisiac effect.   Nadkarni

The *Farmers' Bulletin* (no. 230) issued by the U.S. Department of Agriculture states: Okra, like many other green vegetables, is valued in the diet chiefly because of the nutritionally important minerals it contains. It is a good source of calcium and phosphorus and a fair source of iron. Fresh green okra is also a good source of vitamin A; drying okra reduces the vitamin A content by about half.

In 1951, a university research team announced discovery of okra as a substitute for the plasma in human blood. The substitute was said to have all the advantages of blood plasma and none of its disadvantages.

Nothing more has been heard of the plasma. Okra seems to have slid back into gumbo soup and Creole dishes.

Hieronyma caribaea: Bois D'Amande, Bois Bande

A large tree found in jungles of Trinidad, St. Lucia and other islands of the West Indies where there is plentiful rain. Natives of these islands claim the bark is a powerful aphrodisiac. My informant in Trinidad was an East Indian and in St. Lucia a native.

Honey

The Perfumed Garden gives the following advice: He who feels that he is too weak for coition should drink before going to bed a glassful of thick honey, and eat 20 almonds and 100 grains of the pine tree. He must follow this regime for three days. He may also pulverize onion seed, sift it and mix it afterwards with honey, stirring the mixture well and taking of this mixture while still fasting.

Les Plantes et Les legumes D'Haiti claims honey on bananas makes an "exquisite" aphrodisiac.

Honey most likely was much used by our caveman ancestors to win favors of wild females. Modern man's methods have improved very little.

Hormones

Almost 1,500 years before Christ, Hindu physicians prescribed testicles of sheep to cure impotency. Only in recent years did a scientist discover the male sex hormone testosterone in testicles. It is said that it requires tons of bulls' testicles to produce one one-thousandth of an ounce of the hormone. Testosterone is now made synthetically and prescribed by physicians when they believe male patients require such treatment.

A 1956 report by German veterinarians interested in fodder plants found the flowers of red clover and the flowers and stems of common dandelion enormously rich in estrone hormone. Voisin

Hydrocotyle asiatica

Indian physicians use this herb for rejuvenation.... (It) will improve the colour of the body, youth, memory and give long life.   Nadkarni

Hydrocotyle asiatica aroused considerable interest in 1933 when Chang-li Yun died near Pekin at the purported age of two hundred and fifty-six years old. The fact that he was married twenty four times apparently convinced many that he actually was as old as claimed. Such proof reveals more virility than age.

Hygrophila spinosa

Seeds are given by Hakims with sugar, milk or wine in doses of one to three *dirhem* for impotence. [One dirhem is equal to 3.11 grams.]

A confection of the seeds containing a large number of aphrodisiac, demulcent, nutritious and aromatic stimulant substances has been in use (in India) for impotence, seminal and other debilities.   Nadkarni

Hypoxis aurea: Star-grass
According to Hooper the rootstock swells in water and is mucilaginous.   Its properties are similar to ginseng, being reconstructive, rejuvenating, aphrodisiac, and tonic.   Quisumbing

Stuart alludes to the drug [root] being called 'Brahminical ginseng' on account of its being brought from India. It resembles the Back Musali of the Hindu and Mohammedan physicians. From Sanskrit its name is Ho lun lei t'o, the root of Curculigo orchioides, Gaertn. Its properties are similar to ginseng, being reconstructive, rejuvenating, aphrodisiac, and tonic.

Gardens' Bulletin

Igtnatius beans. (See Strychnos ignatii)

Imperatoria ostruthium: Masterwort
The Decoction of the Root in Wine revives the almost extinct Inclination and Ability to Venery.   Short, 1746

Masterwort is still highly regarded by herbalists in Europe. A German source claims it cleans and detoxicates the blood and stomach; creates appetite; best results used for hardening of arteries. Against the last complaint the masterwort has been a proven agent since ancient times, boiled in wine and drunk before going to bed.

Ipomoea digitata: Fingerleaf morning glory
The powder of the root macerated in its own juice and given with honey ghee is recommended (in India) for use as an aphrodisiac.

Nadkarni

Iron rust
Melampus of Argos, the most ancient Greek physician with whom we are acquainted, is said to have cured one of the Argonauts of sterility, by administering the rust of iron in wine for ten days.   Paris, 1833

Rust of iron steel, nails or other such metal scraps steeped in red wines, were much used in folk practice for tonics and were known as *chalybeates*. Dr. James Ewell gives this recipe in *The Medical Companion or The Family Physician* (1860): Chalybeate Wine - Put rust of steel, one ounce and a half; orange peel and gentian root, each half an ounce, into a bottle of wine. The vessel containing these ingredients is to be exposed to the sun, or near the fire, for three days, and to be repeatedly shaken during this time. This preparation is an excellent stomachic, and agreeable tonic. Dose, for adults, two or three tea-spoonfuls thrice a-day.

Jasminum grandiflorum: Jasmin
Mohammedan writers mention the use of flowers applied as a plaster to the loins, genitals and pubes as an aphrodisiac.

Nadkarni

Jasmine flowers were once much used by Chinese women as a seductive ornament in their hair. Li T'ioa-yiian wrote: "The flower buds, which blossom after dark, are suitable for that very night. After these fragrant buds are placed on the hair, they begin to open. They are brighter and more beautiful under moonlight and they become more fragrant with human warmth, lasting for the whole night and lingering until dawn. Heat can be dispersed by using the flowers as adornment and smelling the fragrance will clear the air for the lungs."

Jugulans regia: Walnut
The meat of the nut has aphrodisiac properties.   Dastur

Walnuts are high in incomplete protein, unsaturated fatty acids, B vitamins, potassium, phosphorus and trace minerals.

Khat. (See Catha edulis)

Leane Bandee'. (See Rhynchosia phaseolides)

Leeks. (See Allium)

Leonurus sibiricus: Siberian motherwort
The seeds are considered to be constructive and aphrodisiac. They are prescribed in loss of virility, and prolonged use promotes fertility.   Stuart

Siberian motherwort contains an essential oil and leonurin. The European species (*L. Cardiaca*) was formerly much used in folk medicine for the heart and nervous conditions of women.

Lepidium sativum: Cress or garden cress
The seed is of vertue like lenny seed, it expelleth wormes, and is ill for women with child, it provoketh termes and Venery.
Langham, 1633

Herb and Seed are acrid, hot, and dry.

It is as powerful an Antiscorbutic as Scurvy Grass, or Water Cresses; therefore Sallads, Diet Drinks, and juices of it, are much in Request in the Spring. The Herb, or juice, cleanse the Reins or Bladder, and provoke Venery.   Short, 1746

A preparation made of seeds, ghee and sugar is a common household remedy (in India) useful as a restorative in general debility. Another invigorating and nutritious tonic to increase the secretion of milk among the lying-in (recently delivered) women is prepared by boiling the seeds in milk so as to form a thin soft mass, and adding to it sufficient sugar or jaggery to make it a confection; this is useful also in seminal debility. Still another invigorating and nutritious diet made of *Lepidium sativum* seeds is prepared by mixing together sufficient quantity of seeds, flowers of tender cocoanut and jaggery and heating them on fire till they melt, mix together and form a molten mass, which is then left to cool and made into large pills and kept for use. Small cakes or balls made for use as aphrodisiacs are made of a mixture of seeds with several other aromatic, nutritious and strength-giving ingredients.   Nadkarni

Licorice. (See **Glycyrrhiza glabra**)

Linaria vulgaris: Toad flax
An old German source mentions this herb as being an effectual remedy to tonic the sexual powers.   Aurand, 1899

This writer found no other record mentioning the above properties. Toad flax is an attractive old-fashioned garden plant. The flowers yield a yellow dye. The herb is used in domestic practice in Europe.

Linum usitatissimum: Flax seed

Being taken largely with pepper and hony made into a cake, it stirreth up lust.   Gerarde, 1636

Flax seed probably is more useful as a poultice than as an aphrodisiac.

Lodoicea sechellarum: Double coconut, coco-de-mer

A remarkably tall palm bearing enormous nuts, each with husk weighing from forty to fifty pounds taking seven to ten years to ripen. An English general wrote in 1882: "Its fruit is shaped like the human heart, the bud or stem which attaches it to the branch like the male organ of generation. When the husk is taken off, the inner double nut is like the belly and thighs of a woman. The male baba and the branch spring from between the thigh-like divisions of the huge leaf stem in a striking way. It is not buried in order to sprout, it is usually placed on the ground where it shoots out a long rod which slits into the plumule and the radicle some ten or twelve feet from the seed, and this forms the bole."

It is said the fruit is taken to India for the harems; its shell is used at the Well of Knowledge at Benares. The insipid-flavored fruit is used in temples of India as aphrodisiac.

Lonicera japonica: Honeysuckle

Prolonged use of flowers, vine and leaves is said to increase vitality and lengthen life.   Stuart

The flowers and leaves have long been used in the Orient to make a cooling tisane. Honeysuckle is native to east Asia. The vine has escaped gardens and now is found in many parts of the United States.

Lotus. (See Nelumbium)

Love Potions and Philtres

Much has been written regarding love potions and they probably have been used since man developed his mind sufficiently to devise means to obtain his ends. The ingredients of such concoctions often ranged from the most loathsome to the most deadly substances man could find. Sometimes there was little difference between a love potion and a poison potion. Albert Magnus' formulae (see *Vinca major*) were particularly rich in revolting and nauseous ingredients. Love potions were used by many of the titled, celebrated, notorious and evil characters throughout history. Brillat-Savarin brought love potions to the gourmet table. He devised special culinary dishes for three types of exhaustion:

No. 1	Due to muscular exertion;
No. 2	Due to mental exhaustion;
No. 3	Due to amorous excesses.

Numbers 1 and 3 are perhaps the most common and overdone; however, they generally recuperate more quickly as they usually induce a relaxed and sound sleep. Number 2 frequently neglects both 1 and 3 and becomes most exhausting as it remains almost constantly with this type worker and interferes with relaxation and sleep.

The efficacy of Brillat-Savarin's recipes were claimed as certain cures for drooping physical faculties, providing the exhausted patient still had a well functioning stomach to tolerate and ingest unusual recipe ingredients.

Lycium chinense: Chinese tea-tree

A common shrub in the northern and western provinces of China. The root is supposed to have a special action on the kidneys and sexual organs.   *Gardens' Bulletin*

The young leaves are consumed as a vegetable.

Madhuca latifolia: Indian butter tree

The flowers mixed with milk are useful in impotence due to general debility; one ounce with eight ounces of fresh milk is the dose.   Nadkarni

Madhuca latifolia is a valuable forest tree of India and seldom cut for timber. The flowers of this tree bloom only at night, then drop to the ground where they are gathered by country people. The flowers are dried and have an agreeable flavor much like pressed figs. People often mix them with other foods, or make them into puddings or candies. Sugar can be extracted from them, and they may be fermented and distilled making an extremely strong drink.

The fleshy fruits of Indian butter tree contain from one to four seeds, highly valued as a food. The outer coat of the fruit is eaten as a vegetable, and the inner portion is dried and ground into flour. A thick oil is obtained from the kernels which is used for cooking or making soap and candles.

Maerua angolensis

In North Nigeria the fruit is used by young men as a love charm, mixed with *tozali* (galena, or so-called "antimony") and rubbed in the eyelids it renders them irresistible to girls. The plant is attractive as an ornamental shrub for the garden, especially in the drier regions.   Dalziel

The leaves of *Maerua* are eaten as a vegetable by Africans and the roots of another species (*M. pedunculosa*) are eaten in times of scarcity.

Several years ago a national magazine had an interesting article about elephants in South Africa getting tipsy after eating the "merula" fruit which they are very fond of. Another magazine had an item regarding the conviction of a young South African accused of sexually assaulting two women nine times in rapid succession. At the trial, the accused claimed that he lost control of himself after eating a number of the fruit from the "murula" tree. This writer searched in vain through a number of botanical books and found no record of "murula" fruit. Is it possible the magazine items referred to *Maerua?*

Mammea americana: Mamey

A beautiful fruit tree native to the West Indies. Primitive Caribbean tribes considered the fruit sacred and very potent, which only the men were permitted to eat. In the French West Indies the fragrant flowers are used to make a liqueur known as "eau de creole" or "creme de creole." The fruit is sometimes sliced and served with wine or with sugar and cream. It is also prepared as a sauce, preserves or jam.

Mandragora officinarum: Mandrake

This plant should not be confused with American mandrake (Podophyllum peltatum).

Mandragora was used since ancient times by Greek, Roman, and Arabian physicians. Dioscorides, a physician in Nero's army, described the hypnotic effect of a wine decoction made with mandragora and commonly used by physicians of his time. It served as an anesthetic for surgical operations and also to stupefy criminals and Christians sentenced to death. Mandragora was much used in love potions and sexual orgies by the Romans and throughout the Middle Ages. It was believed to excite the amorous propensity and remedy female sterility. Mandragora's ancient history as an aphrodisiac lingered on until superseded by new aphrodisiacs brought by traders from the Orient and the New World.

Marijuana   (See Cannabis sativa)

Marjoram.   (See Origanum majorana)

64

Matricaria chamomilla: German chamomile

Chamomile tea applied to the genitals has a powerful stimulating effect.   Nadkarni

This writer has studied countless Materia Medica records for more than half a century and never found the above ascribed to German Chamomile elsewhere.

The flowers have been used since ancient times externally as a fomentation or warm moist application for earache, neuralgic pains and colic in babies. The infusion is very popular in Europe for young and old.

Mentha species: Mints

All mints, greene or dry, are good for the stomacke, and also the distilled water, to help digestion, to avoid the hicket [hiccup], lothing and choller, especially used in sawces: it provoketh lust, and comforteth all members, and the smell of it comforteth the brains and memory.   Langham, 1633

M. spicata: Spearmint   (See also **Mentha spicata** in **Anaphrodisiacs.**)

Spearmint is a provoker of venery.   Monroe, 1824

Meum athamanticum: Spignel, baldmony or bawdwort

The roots of Meon (Spignel), boyled in water and drunke, mightily open the stoppings of the kidnies, and bladder, provoke urine and bodily lust.   Gerarde, 1636

Spignel is a glorious Plant to cold, phlegmatic, and cachectic constitutions, a Kind of Treacle or panacea, from its much contained exalted Oil, and volatile or essential Salt; it therefore affects the Heads of the Choleric or Sanguine, if taken too long, or too large Doses. The root expels Wind, and discusses Flatulency or Belchings; it powerfully provokes Urine and

Menses, is excellent in Hysterics, green-Sickness, Catarrhs, Gripes, and facilitates Venery much. Short, 1746

Spignel is a very aromatic perennial common in the meadows of the Alps.

Momordica balsamina: Balsam-pear
Dalziel mentions the root of this vine is sometimes an ingredient in aphrodisiac prescriptions.

M. charantia
The seeds benefit the breath and invigorate the male principle.
Stuart

Moringa oleifera: Horseradish tree
Flowers are sometimes boiled with milk and the preparation is used as an aphrodisiac. Nadkarni

Horseradish tree is common throughout the West Indies. The young leaves are used as greens and the root is used like our garden variety as the flavor remarkably resembles this condiment. The seeds are the source of oil of bene used for lubricating watches and delicate instruments.

Mucuna (Stizolobium) giganteum: Sea-bean or great oxeye bean
The seeds are sometimes used as watch charms; powdered, they are used as an aphrodisiac. This plant is widely spread in Polynesia, tropical Asia and eastern Australia. Grows on the edge of the forests and in thickets along the roadside, sometimes climbing over high trees. Safford

M. pruriens
The hairs of the pod, known as cowhage in medicine are mixed with honey or molasses and given as a vermifuge. The powdered

66

seeds are used in India as an aphrodisiac, and the young green pods are cooked and eaten as a vegetable.

Safford

A compound of powder made of the seeds, and of the fruits of *Tribulus terrestris* taken in equal parts is recommended to be administered in doses of 1 drachm with sugar and tepid milk as an aphrodisiac.

Susruta

According to Dalziel the fruits and sometimes the whole plant of *Tribulus terrestris* are used as a diuretic and are said to be valuable in bladder troubles.

Another preparation known Vanari Vatika is recommended in Bhavaprakash. It is made by boiling 32 tolas [5760 grains] of the seeds [or litres] in 4 seers of cow's milk till the milk becomes thick; seeds are then decorticated [husks removed] and pounded, then fried in ghee and made into a confection with double their weight of sugar. The mass is then divided into balls which are kept steeped in honey. Dose is about a tola. This is one of the best aphrodisiacs.

Nadkarni

Muira-puama: Potency-wood
A shrubby plant found mainly in regions near the Amazon River. The root and woody stems have a reputation for being a powerful aphrodisiac in Brazil. It is an ingredient of several widely advertised sexual impotence formulas in Germany. According to German researchers Muira-puama contains an aromatic resin, two acids, an unknown crystalline substance, tannin, muirapuanine, and an amorphous bitter substance.

Mushrooms. (See **Tuber**)

67

Musk

Genuine musk is derived from the glands of the male musk-deer of the mountains of the Himalayan ranges.

Davenport wrote that when musk is taken internally it is said by many physicians to be almost equal to ambergris for its aphrodisiacal qualities. Externally applied, this substance produces very singular phenomena. Weickard says that by means of this drug he resuscitated the genital power in a man who had nearly completed his eightieth year.

Myrtus communis: Myrtle

The leaves mixed with cordial syrups is a good cordial and inclines those that drink it to be very amorous. The myrtle was used in the composition prepared for the most intimate toilet of Venus and probably from its association with the goddess has always been regarded as a love tonic.

Leyel

Nandina domestica: Nandina

An evergreen shrub with beautiful red berries found growing on the hills of China. Medicinally, the branches and leaves are reputed to check discharges, drive away sleepiness, strengthen the tendons, benefit the breath, prolong life, prevent hunger, and keep off old age. They are also prescribed for colds. The seeds have about the same virtues, and they are said to strengthen virility and improve the complexion. The congee, made with leaves, has similar virtues, to which are added the nourishing qualities of the rice. Stuart

The Nandina is widely planted in China for its glossy luxuriant foliage and for its white flowers produced on large showy panicles followed by clusters of shining berries. The plant does not tolerate cold climate.

Nasturtium officinale: Watercress

The seeds have tonic, alterative, aphrodisiac, stimulant and aperient properties.

Dastur

Watercress, parsley, dandelion greens and alfalfa herb are probably the greatest land vegetable sources of vitamins, minerals and trace elements.

Quantities of watercress are grown in Trinidad and India to help supplement nutritional deficiencies of vegetarian diets.

Nelubium nucifera: Chinese, East Indian lotus or sacred lotus.

The lotus is one of the most beautiful of all Asiatic flowers and the most sacred plant of Buddhism. Its religious significance transcends the natural range of the plant according to Dr. Li. The sacred lotus is mentioned in Tibetan mythology and the flower is a symbol on temples, charms and amulets. All parts of the plant are used in China as food and medicine. The marble size seeds were once an expensive luxury reserved for the rich. They are eaten raw, candied, roasted, boiled or ground in flour. They are considered nourishing, beneficial in preserving bodily health and strength as well as being aphrodisiac. The rootstock, which resemble large links of sausages, is boiled and eaten sliced or reduced to an aromatic and sweet flour resembling arrowroot. The flour is held to be a nutritious tonic, increasing mental faculties and quieting the spirits. It is also believed to be of value in the treatment of diarrhoea, dysentery and diseases of the chest. Like arrowroot, the flour is used for infants, convalescent and the aged.

A yellow flowering lotus (*Nelumbo lutea*) was much used as a food and medicine by American Indians.

Nettle. (See Urtica dioica)

69

Newbouldia laevis

A familiar live fence and boundry tree in Africa. The roots and leaves are believed to have aphrodisiac properties. Dalziel

Oats. (See Avena sativa)

Okra. (See Hibiscus esculentus)

Onions. (See Allium cepa)

Ophiopogon japonicus: Mai-tung or mak-tung

This plant grows throughout China, Mongolia and Japan. It is cultivated near Peking and in the province of Chekiang. The candied tubers are eaten as a medicine and are regarded as tonic and aphrodisiac. *Gardens' Bulletin*

Orchis latifolia, O. maculata, O. mascula, O. morio: Salep; ancient name satyrion

All the kindes of orchis are accounted to procure bodily lust, as well the flowers distilled, as the rootes prepared.

Parkinson, 1629

Dioscorides wrote that it was reported, That if men do eat of the great full or fat roots of these kinds of Dogs stones (Orchis), they cause them to beget male children; and if women eat of the lesser dry or barren root which is withered or shriveled, they shall bring forth females. These are some Doctours opinions only. It is further reported, That in Thessalia the women give the full and tender root to be drunk in goats milk, to move bodily lust, and the dry to restrain the same. Gerarde, 1636

O. morio: Salep

The Roots are accounted a provocative and a Stimulus to Venery, and a Strengthener of the genital Parts, and help Conception, and for those Purposes are a chief Ingredient in the

70

Electuarium Diasatyrium. The only Officinal Preparation is the
Aforesaid Electuary.   J. Miller, 1722

With the Turks salep is in great celebrity on account of the
restorative qualities which they imagine it to possess. It is much
recommended as nutritive food for persons recovering from
illness; and in a particular manner as a part of the stores of every
ship about to sail into distant climates. It not only possesses the
property of yielding an invaluable nutriment, and in a great
measure of concealing the saline taste of seawater, but is likewise
of essential service against the sea-scurvy. When it is stated that
an ounce of this powder and an ounce of portable soup, dissolved
in two quarts of boiling water, will form a jelly capable of
affording sustenance to one man for a day, the utility of salep will
be further seen as a means of preventing famine at sea for an
infinitely longer time than any other food of equal bulk.
                                                   Bingley, 1816

The root yields a large quantity of mucilage to water and, on
boiling even with 40 parts of water, forms a thick jelly which is
highly nutritious and wholesome. It forms one of the best articles
of diet for weak or convalescent persons. For this purpose,
powder of salep roots is the best for use; usually cooked with
milk in the proportion of 1 teaspoon to a tea cupful of milk.

It is given in all forms of wasting disease. Salep has long been
esteemed in India as a great restorative and invigorator and a
tonic aphrodisiac in diseases characterized by weakness or loss of
sexual powers. A decoction of the leaves of sacred basil with the
addition of a little cardamon powdered and about a tola [180
grains] of salep powdered, makes a nourishing and aphrodisiac
drink.   Nadkarni

The orchis works direct wonders for weak children. The
debilitated and weak body is quickly strengthened; not only

children, but adults also are benefited by it. Furthermore orchis root is recommended for diarrhea, inflammation ailments and to strengthen sexual nerves of women as well as men. For this evil one must drink the infusion three times a day.   Rogler

Origanum majorana: Marjoram

Marjoram was proved by Dr. Cessoles on himself and two young women; and the symptoms of the proving showed a distinct relation of the sexual organs, which clinical experience has verified and expanded. All kinds of sexual excitement, in females especially, have been remedied by Origanum. The sexual symptoms were developed chiefly in the female provers, and were these: Sadness followed by joyfulness and thoughts of marriage. Lascivious dreams, increased desire for coitus. Swelling and itching of nipples and pains in breasts. The additional symptoms in the Schema are cured symptoms collected by Hering. I have frequently verified the power of Origanum in morbid sexual excitement in both sexes.   Clarke

In moderate doses, extract of *Origanum majorana* appears to operate contrary to the above statement. (See **Origanum majorana** in **Anaphrodisiacs.**)

Orobanche ammophyla or O. major

The ancients thought that this plant sprang up from the semen dropped on the ground by wild stallions, somewhat similar to the supposed origin of Balenophera, another orobancaceous plant. Its virtues seem to be tonic in all of the wasting diseases and injuries, as well as aphrodisiac, promoting fertility in women and curing impotence in men. It is used in spermatorrhea, menstrual difficulties, gonorrhea, and all forms of difficulties of the genital organs. The Lieh-tang (another species) has similar virtues, but is specially recommended in impotence. Both the plant (Orobanche) and root are eaten either raw or cooked with meat.   Stuart

Orobanche is a parasitic plant.

Panax ginseng: Chinese ginseng

Chinese ginseng is the most esteemed and celebrated drug in Oriental Materia Medica. No other panacea has been attributed with so many properties. It is believed to remove all fatigue either of body or mind; dissolve humours; cure pulmonary diseases; strengthen the stomach and, most of all, increase the vital powers, and promote life to old age. Chinese at death's door use ginseng in belief the root would hold off the grim reaper long enough to enable the person to settle earthly affairs and bid friends and loved ones farewell.

Many medicines after an elapse of time are discarded, neglected or pigeonholed to a specific us. Ginseng differs completely. The root appears to gather more virtues with years. A modern Korean advertisement adds new claims for the panacea. The manufacturer advertises its products with a handsome colored brochure showing on the cover an exotic old Oriental holding a strange plant while the back cover has a photo of a tall building evidently where ginseng is processed or given special treatment. The brochure contains no picture of the genuine plant or farms where it is grown. The following are the medical claims made by the Korean company:

Main pharmacological actions are:
1   It acts as a rejuvenator and reactivates the endocrine glands.
2   It strengthens the heart and nervous system.
3   It increases the body's hormones.
4   It stimulates metabolism, physical growth, and prevents fatigue and ageing phenomenon.
5   It strengthens resistance against various stresses, ailments and pathogens through stimulation of cerebrocortical functions.

6   It helps in increasing the production of blood cells by stimulating hematopoietic organ and promoting blood circulation.

7   It promotes appetite and digestion, maintaining normal body condition.

Efficacy:

General weakness, anemia, sexual decline, mental exhaustion, mental and physical fatigue, high blood pressure, before and after disease, before and after delivery, indigestion, diabetes, etc.

Old Chinese revered ginseng especially because the root could be taken regardless of age or physical condition without reaction or shock to the system even when taken over long periods of time.   Li Yutang, noted author and philosopher wrote, "I am willing to give personal testimony as to its [ginseng] being the most energy giving tonic known to mankind, distinguished by the slowness and gentleness of its action."   Slowness of action apparently does not fit with the trend of modern times.   In this jet-age people want fast action, disregarding the consequences or hoping another wonder drug will cure the reactions of the first one.   A recent issue of a well known American magazine reveals how two potentially toxic drugs were added to ginseng pills produced by a pharmaceutical company in Hong Kong.   One ingredient was phenylbutazone, a popular drug used for certain arthritic conditions.   The other ingredient was aminopyrine, which can alter the white blood cells so they become impotent and unable to protect the body from infection.   The U.S. Food and Drug Administration officials believed the drugs were added to give the ginseng pills a physiological discernible effect.

There is now a tremendous demand for ginseng, and it appears inconceivable that a plant so rare could possibly supply the market, especially since the root is "only grown in a limited area requiring full six years of ceaseless attention and immeasurable care." (Excerpt from Korean advertisement).   Korean ginseng is

74

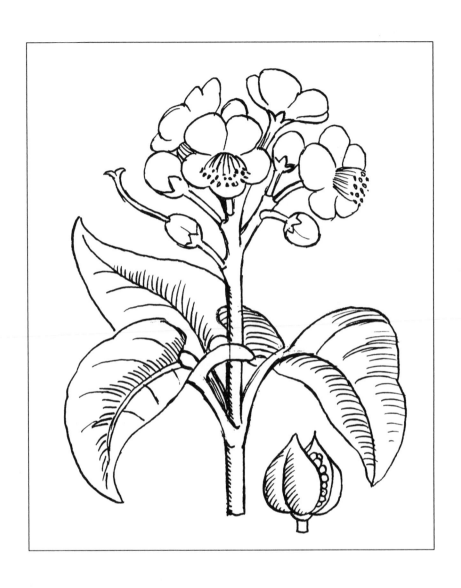

ANATTO
(*Bixa orellana*)
See page 28

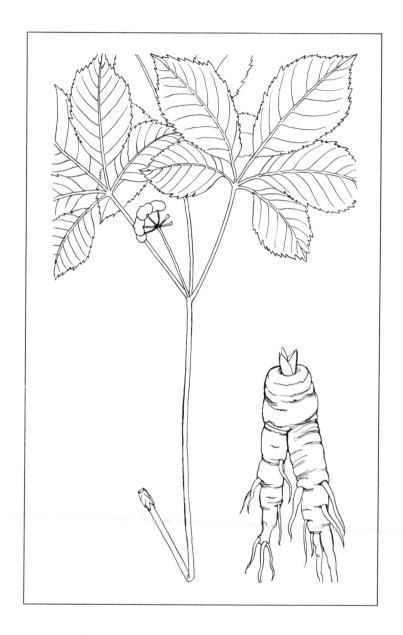

AMERICAN GINSENG
(*Panax quinquefolia*)
See page 75

now offered in two colors and a variety of forms, including instant tea and chewing gum.

Panax quinquefolia: American ginseng

It is interesting to note that the American Indians did not regard this plant as an important medicinal. The root was sometimes used by early settlers and colonists for minor conditions. American ginseng was considered inferior to the Chinese variety and often substituted for the real article after getting special treatment. Perhaps the first authoritative mention of American ginseng was by J.R. Coxe, M.D. in his book *The American Dispensatory* (1818). The doctor wrote, "The Americans disregard it because it is found plentifully in their woods." *The Dispensatory of the United States*, by G. B. Wood, M.D. and F. Bache, M.D. (1858) states, "It [American ginseng] is little more than a demulcent, and in this country is not employed as a medicine." Nearly a century later a well known botanical journal made a similar statement: "The root is actually little more than a demulcent, and today in America it is rarely used as a curative." Apparently little or no American research has been done on our native ginseng to change the rubber-stamp opinion. Regardless of medical judgement, the supply of American ginseng often falls far short of the demand.

Pandanus odoratissimus: Fragrant screwpine

The root pulverized in milk is used (in India) internally in sterility and threatened abortion.   Nadkarni

Pandanus species

The young flower spikes boiled in milk are used as a love potion by the Malaysians.   Burkill

Pansinystalia yohimbe: Yohimbe

A tall tree native of Africa. The bark has a reputation in Cameroons as an aphrodisiac, and yields two alkaloids, yohimbine

75

and yohimbinine. The former is poisonous and exerts a local anaesthetic action like cocaine, but with dilating the pupil and without harmful effect on the cornea. It has been used as an aphrodisiac mainly in veterinary medicine. Yohimbinine has no physiological action. (Henry, *Plant Alkaloides*, 394-395, under *Corynanthe Johimbe*). Dalziel

Like Muira-puama, yohimbe is an ingredient of formulas offered in Continental Europe as an aphrodisiac and nerve stimulant.

Pastinaca sativa: Parsnip
The boiled roots of parsnip may be eaten with good sweet butter, vinegar, or lime-juice, or juice of lemons and mustard. They are very palatable and nourishing, restore in consumption, open, attenuate and cleanse the bowels, fasten the body, breed seed plentifully, and provoke to venery. The seed taken in powder to a dram, or a strong decoction thereof expels wind, provokes urine and lust, and gives present ease in the colic.
Salmon, 1710

Pega palo. (See **Rhynchosia**)

Penianthus patulinervis
The roots and twigs are used as chewsticks, chewed or prepared in decoction by the people of Sierra Leone and Ivory Coast, as an aphrodisiac, and in Ashanti to cure cough.   Dalziel

Perfumes. (See **Rosa** and **Jasminum**)

Persea americana: Avocado
Standley declares a large number of therapeutic uses are reported for the plant. The pulp is credited as having aphrodisiac properties. Quisumbing

Fray Francisco Ximenez, a follower of Hernandez, says: "The pulp awakens a great sexual appetite and increases the semen."

Martinez

Avocados are an excellent source of potassium, phosphorus, sulphur, magnesium and other elements.

Petroselinum hortense: Parsley
The seed taken aforehand, withstandeth drunkennesse, it stirreth up women to conception. Langham, 1633

Parsley is one of the oldest known herbs and still highly regarded in Europe. In the United States it is used mainly as a flavoring herb or as a garnish which is generally tossed aside. The herb is particularly rich in vitamin A which helps prevent night blindness and, among other things, in keeping the skin supple and youthful. Parsley is also rich in vitamin C and appreciable amounts of vitamin B factors as well as minerals and trace elements. The infusion of the herb is an excellent diuretic and said also to give relief or ease arthritic pains.

Phoenix dactylifera: Date palm
Date is very nutritious, its infusion in milk is very nourishing and restorative. An infusion of the fresh fruit in water is useful for relieving alcoholic intoxication. Dastur

Physalis angulata: Ground cherry
In North Nigeria the plant is used by women as an infusion drunk in childbirth; the fruit crushed with milk is a remedy for sterility. Dalziel

P. minima: Cape gooseberry
Nadkarni reports that the fruit is said to infuse vigor in a worn-out system and offset premature decay. Dymock tells us

that in the Konkan the plant is made into a paste with rice water and applied to restore flaccid breasts.   Quisumbing

In Guam the fruit is eaten by the natives; it forms a good salad, when raw, or made into a dulce. Chickens are fond of it.
                                                                                    Safford

P. alkekengi: Winter cherry, strawberry tomato
This variety contains an alkaloid and bitters physalin. The berries are said to contain more vitamin C than lemons.

Pimpinella anisum: Anise, Aniseed
The seeds eaten plentifully provoketh lust, and doe breed milk.
                                                                        Langham, 1633

The seed wasteth and consumeth winde, and is good against belchings and upbraidings of the stomacke, allaieth gripings of the belly, provoketh urine gently, maketh abundance of milke, and stirreth bodily lust.   Gerarde, 1636

Ancient Rome was notorious for its debauches and feasts. At weddings they made a cake called "mustacea" which consisted of meal, aniseed and other aromatics. Romans ate the wedding cake to remove or prevent indigestion caused by overeating at the marriage entertainment. Many modern wedding cakes decorated with synthetic colors and flavors would add to the misery of over-indulgences.

Pinus species: Pine sap
The same is good against the stone in the kidnies, and against frettings of the bladder, and scalding of urine, for it allayeth the sharpnesse, mitigateth pain, and gently provoketh urine: moreover it increaseth milke and seed, and therefore it also provoketh fleshly lust.   Gerarde, 1636

The seeds of "Stone Pine" (native of Italy) are nourishing and aphrodisiac.   Whitlaw, 1829

Piper betle: Betel pepper
The leaves are aromatic, aphrodisiac and exhilarant.   Dastur

P. cubeba: Cubebs
Dumas has told us that Hindus steep the dried berries in wedding wine when the groom is older than forty.

P. guineense: West African pepper, Guinea cubebs
The leaves taken with food are supposed to improve chances of conception.   Dalziel

Pistacia vera: Pistache or pistachio
The bark of the tree is said to be strengthening to the female principle.   Stuart

Almond-like fruits are a source of pistachio oil. The oil is used to flavor sauces, foods and confectionery.

Plantago major: Common plantain
The drug [seed] is good for wasting diseases in male and female, promotes the secretion of the semen, and therefore conduces to fertility.   Stuart

Plantain is a lawn weed once believed to follow the white man wherever he goes. It is a valuable plant in folk medicine. (See *American Folk Medicine* by Clarence Meyer.)

Polygala reinii
The root is considered warming and tonic. It strengthens the bones and sinews, quiets the five viscera, is tonic to the centres, increasing the will power and benefits the breath.
Gardens' Bulletin

Polygonum multiflorum

Fabulous stories are told in the Pen ts'as (Chinese Herbal, 1596) of the powers of this root: to give long life, increase vigour, and promote fertility.   *Gardens' Bulletin*

Psoralea corylifolia

The plant is native of India, and is met with in the south and west China. The flat, oval or slightly reniform, black one-seeded legumes are about 3 to 4 millimeters long, and often retain the persistent, five-lobed, calyx. They have an aromatic odor, and a biter, aromatic flavor. They are regarded as highly aphrodisiac and tonic to the genital organs, and are prescribed in all forms of sexual impotency.   Threatened abortion, the discomforts of pregnancy, insufficient erections, polyuria, and incontinence of urine in children, are difficulties for which the drug is administered.   Stuart

In India the seeds are regarded as aphrodisiac.   Dastur

Rhinoceros horn

Rhino horn is in great demand as an aphrodisiac in India, China and Southeast Asia. No amount of medical proof can change the Asian's faith in its efficacy. Chinese believe a love potion of the ground-up horn will turn a shy fellow into a Romeo, and make he-men out of weak men. Rhinos are threatened with extinction because of such beliefs.

In South America, Indians of the Guianas esteemed the horny hoofs of another animal. (See **Tapir.**)

Rhynchosia phaseolides: Pega palo, leane bandee

Almost 500 years after Juan Ponce de Leon left Santa Domingo to search for the Fountain of Youth, another legend originated from the old city. This time the legend came from the bars of Santa Domingo as well as bars in Port-au-Prince, capital of Haiti, which shares the island of Hispaniola. Wondrous virility powers were attributed to a vine found on this island. In Dominican Republic it is known as pega palo, in Haiti as liane bandee. This writer's information was gleaned from Ceasare Montrez, bartender in the hotel Citadella perched on a mountain overlooking Port-au-Prince. Montrez's direction was to steep one inch of the stalk of liane bandee in a bottle of rum for one week. Doses were a jiggerful three times per day. Montrez warned overdosing was dangerous. He knew a Haitian who took too much and it eventually killed him because, as he explained, "it never went down." Another Haitian informant told this writer, liane bandee was scarce in Haiti and only grew on the mountain of Kenscoff. The specimen shown resembled a dark-green electric extension cord with three or four strands of wire-like vines flattened together. The plant is not confined to Hispaniola as botanists have reported it in the high hills of Bayamon, Puerto Rico, and in other Antilles, Panama, Brazil, and the Galapagos Islands. Apparently there is no other record of the vine being used as an aphrodisiac. *Rhynchosia phaseolides* was exploited more in Santo Domingo than in Haiti. One of the first billboard signs this writer saw upon arriving at the airport was that of the so-called rejuvenator. American tourists carried the news of pega palo to bars of Miami and New York, whence the "great" news spread like wildfire to bars of other cities. The "fires" were quickly extinguished by several states and the United States Department of Agriculture.

Rocket. (See **Eruca sativa**)

Rosa moschata: Musk-scented rose
   The variety is cultivated in India for the production of attar. It is aphrodisiac.   Nadkarni

Attar of rose becomes a psychological aphrodisiac to the male when the perfume is artfully used by a voluptuous young female. The mental factor is greatly enhanced by clothes--better no clothes, sensuous movements, soft music, titillating foods, and pleasant surrounds. The combination is generally sufficient to motivate amatory notions even in exhausted old males if a spark of sex life remains.

Rubus species: Chinese raspberry
The Chinese raspberry is found in the uplands of the central and western provinces, where there are about sixty species. Dried raspberries are supposed to benefit respiration, give vigour to the body, and prevent hair from falling off.   They have tonic, restorative, and aphrodisiac properties.   *Gardens' Bulletin*

Ruta graveolens: Rue
Rue provoketh lust in women.   Langham, 1633

(See **Ruta** in **Anaphrodisiacs**.)

Saffron. (See **Crocus sativus**)

Salep. (See **Orchis**)

Salvadore oleoides: Mustard tree
The sweet fruit is believed in India to have aphrodisiac properties however "fruits eaten singly cause tingling and small ulcers in the mouth."   Nadkarni

Shoots and young leaves are eaten as salad, and as fodder for camels. A vegetable salt is derived from the ash of the plant.

Salt
Ancient Greeks believed all life had its origin in the sea. They glorified the belief that Aphrodite (or Venus), the goddess of love, arose into life from the foam of sea waves. Ferdinand Gomez (1388-1457), celebrated physician, asserted that women who indulged in salt became more salacious. Prof. J. Ranke (1878)

wrote: "In the blood man carried the sea, so to speak, in his body about with him, which bathes and nourishes all the cells. Not a single living cell of the total organism can exist even for the shortest moment without the regular interchange with this vital fluid," salt sea.

In more recent times a well-known medical columnist extols the water-soluble properties of trace elements found in sea water. The doctor mentions Ponce de Leon sailing with his galleon over a veritible sea of health-giving-waters in his search for the Fountain of Youth.

The fluid around the cells of the human body that constitutes thirty percent of it is essentially diluted sea water. This is believed to be the result of life's origin in the oceans billions of years ago. For maintenance of our internal environment, it is suggested our dietary intake of minerals should duplicate the mineral elements found in sea water, plus certain elements for specific needs.

Salvia haematodes: Bloodveined sage

Root contains fat, tannic acid and a bitter crystalline alkaloid "Bahmanine." It is tonic, astringent and aphrodisiac, and one of the ingredients of various compound astringent decoctions and aphrodisiac confections which are largely prescribed (in India) for seminal debility.   Nadkarni

S. officinalis: Garden sage

It is good for women with child to eate of this herbe, for as Aetius saith, it closeth the matrix, causeth the fruite to live, and strengtheneth the same. Sage causeth women to be fertill, wherefore in times past the people of Egypt, after a great mortalitie and pestilence, constrained their women to drinke the juice thereof, to cause them the sooner to conceive, and to bring forth store of children, which are the blessing of God.

Dodoens, 1586

Garden sage is one of our oldest medicinals and still much used in folk practice. (See *American Folk Medicine*). Garden sage also is much used to impart its healthy aroma and flavor to tomato dishes, poultry stuffing, soups, herb butter, cheese, sausage and fatty meats such as pork, duck and goose. The pungency of sage enables the stomach to help digest fat meats more easily.

S. plebeia: East Indian sage
Seeds are demulcent and nutritive. In India they are used for seminal weakness and to promote sexual powers.   Nadkarni

S. sclarea: Clary sage
The seed poudered and drunke with wind, stirreth up bodily lust.   Gerarde, 1636

A dram of powdered Clary taken inwardly provokes venery.
Salmon, 1710

Hormium (old Latin name for clary sage) in Greek means to rush, or be carried with force, because by its force it stimulates and violently increases the venereal appetite.   P. Miller, 1737

Both seed and leaves taken in wine excite venery. The herb put into ale either stupifies the drinker, or makes him outrageous.
Short, 1746

Sarsaparilla. (See Smilax)

Satureja hortensis: Summer savory
The use of Saverie in meats, doth long preserve the body in health; it helpeth swellings and gripings in the body, it helpeth digestion, it expelleth the superfluittes of the stomacke, provoketh urine and termes, and sharpeneth the weak sight that is dulled with evill moisture, moveth carnell lust, quickeneth the wits or brains.   Langham, 1633

Summer Savory. The infusion is the warmest and most stimulating of garden herbs.   Hand, 1820

The herb is resolvent, exciting, expelling, stomachic, emmenagogue, aphrodisiac. The herb and seeds in debility of stomach, and for procreation.   Whitlaw, 1829

Satyrion. (See Orchis)

Saussurea lappa: Costus
The root is regarded as a tonic, and is still used by the Malays. It is held to be aphrodisiac, which in the East is the chief way of estimating tonic properties.   Burkill

The root contains the alkaloid saussurine; for medicinal requirements the root is collected during September and October; it is reputed to be aphrodisiac.   Dastur

The essential oil (*Saussurea lappa*) is excreted in the urine and during its passage through the urethra it may produce a certain amount of irritation giving rise to aphrodisiac effects.   Nadkarni

Uphof wrote the root of costus has been used since remote times and much of it is now exported to China and the Red Sea area. It is used in perfumery, blending well with khus-khus, rose geranium, sandalwood, patchouly and giving bouquets of the Oriental type perfumes. Also used in incenses and fumigants. It is said that hairwash made of costus root has a reputation for turning gray hair black.

Saw palmetto. (See Serenoa serrulata)

Sea foods
Fresh fish, shell-fish, and oysters have a reputation of being aphrodisiac, which they have obtained simply because they are

highly nutritive and readily digestible. It is indeed possible that sea foods have some peculiar tonic influence, owing to a small portion of phosphorus which they usually contain, that chemical element having a powerful effect in maintaining nervous force. Icelanders and sea-coast tribes, subsisting principally on fish, much of it eaten raw, are often reported in books of travel to be unusually salacious.   Napheys, 1871

Octopus, cuttlefish and caviar are also reputed to be aphrodisiacs.   Dr. Thomas Venner especially recommended shrimps. He wrote, "Pranes and Shrimps are of one and the same nature: for goodnesse of meat they excell all other shell-fish: they are of a very good temperature and substance, of a most sweet and pleasant taste, not of hard concoction, and of excellent nourishment. By reason of their moyst and calorificall nature, they propitiate *Venus:* they are convenient of every age and constitution of body, with this proviso, that the stomack be not weak."

The following anecdote relative to the property in seafood is related by Hecquet: "Sultan Saladin, wishing to ascertain the extent of the continence of the dervishes [Moslem orders living in monasteries or wandering as friars], took two of them into his palace, and, during a certain space of time, had them fed upon the most succulent food. In a short time all traces of their self-inflicted severities were effaced, and their *embonpoint* began to re-appear. In this state he gave them two Odalisques [female slaves or harem concubines] of surpassing beauty, for the two holy men came forth from the ordeal as pure as the diamond of Bejapore.

"The Sultan still kept them in his palace, and, to celebrate their triumph, caused them to live upon a diet equally *recherce,* but consisting entirely of fish. A few days afterwards they were again subjected to the united powers of youth and beauty, but this time nature was too strong, and the two happy cenobites forgot, in

86

the arms of voluptuousness, their vows of continence and
chastity."   Davenport, 1869

   In Japan about one hundred people die every year from eating
a gourmet's delight known as the puffer fish or fugu. The ovaries
and liver of the puffer contain the deadly poison tetrodotoxin.
One ounce is said to be capable of killing fifty-six thousand
diners! The puffer is ambrosial best in winter. It is served raw in
very thin slices or stewed with vegetables. Sometimes it is drunk
as a potion of hot sake with puffer testes that reputedly enhances
virility. Fish livers contain more vitamin A than any other known
food.
   In the Orient shark fins are also much esteemed as a food and
aphrodisiac. In Europe the eel is also believed to give strength
where it is needed. King Henry IV of France instructed his chef
to keep a potful of eel saute hot on the stove for every hour of the
day for occasions when he felt his flesh to be weak while his
spirit was willing. It is said Mme. Thevenin served dishes of eel
and truffles in her highly regarded brothel.
   In the West Indies the conch was a favorite food of the Carib
Indians and now the former descendants of salves. Conch meat is
valued for its strengthening powers. The following recipe was
said to be an octogenarian rejuvenator: "Remove the rubbery
inhabitant from its shell. Some cooks wash it with soap to get rid
of the grease, tenderize by rubbing or wrapping with papaya leaf.
Pour boiling water over it and rinse. Cut in small pieces or keep
it whole. Saute with 'piment', onion and garlic and a little
vinegar and water. Tomato sauce may be added or parsley."
   The eggs of sea turtles are also reputed to be aphrodisiac.
Sea-egg or sea urchin, according to Collymore, provides
Barbadians with one of their most delectable dishes, and which,
according to popular lore, is the case of the islanders virility and
fertility. Sea-eggs are eaten raw, lightly boiled or fried with
onions like an omelette. Whether raw, fried or boiled, a squeeze

of lime enhances the dish. The flavor of sea-egg is sweet and delicate, somewhat like that of the yolk of chicken egg.

This writer's Bahamian gardener told him the natives of "de islands" rarely eat lobsters because they make one lazy the following day. The words lazy or exhausted apparently have the same meaning among some Bahamians.

Schizandra chinensis

The fruits are called "the drug with five tastes or flavours." The skin and pulp are sweet and sour, the kernels are pungent and bitter, the whole drug has a saltish taste. Tonic, aphrodisiac, pectoral, and lenitive properties are ascribed to the drug by the Malayas. *Gardens' Bulletin*

The Chinese use this plant in much the same way. Stuart, however, adds "the Chinese unwisely reject the branches, which yield a mucilaginous decoction, efficacious in dysentery, gonorrhoea, and coughs."

Schizandra is an ornamental vine often grown for its handsome bright green foliage, pinkish white flowers and scarlet berries.

Scrophularia oldhami: Figwort

The root when dried becomes purplish black and sweetish to the taste. Like the true ginseng root it is considered a potent restorative; preparations of this root specially acting on the kidneys. *Gardens' Bulletin*

The roots are regarded as cooling, diuretic, tonic and restorative, and are prescribed in fevers, malaria, typhoid, scrophulous glands, galactorrhoea, and leucorrhoea. Stuart

Schrophularia nodosa, S. lanceolata and S. marylandica were highly regarded in folk practice.

Securinega virosa
Caius states that in Rhodesia the root is used as an aphrodisiac. Bailey reported some varieties are cultivated and have proved fairly hardy at Arnold Arboretum.

Semecarpus anacardium: Oriental cashew nut, marking nut
It is believed in India that the drug [fruit] taken in small but gradually increasing doses in the winter, makes one free from cough and colds and senile degenerations. Dr. H.C. Sen states that he has seen a man 108 years old who has been using a confection of the drug for many years during winter and that the man is yet fairly strong, his hair has not turned grey and his teeth have not fallen out, although his power of hearing is very deficient. The fruit is reputed to be aphrodisiac.   Nadkarni

The juice of Oriental cashew is used with lime water to make an ink used on cloth. The oil of the nuts is used in India for protection against white ants and for floor dressing. Nuts are also used for tanning. The cashew nuts we know and consume in great quantities when roasted is *Anacardium occidentale*, native of tropical America.

Serenoa serrulata: Saw palmetto
Highly recommended for all wasting diseases. It is a remarkable strength builder, and a great restorer of lost energy and vitality.   *The Famous Book of Herbs, 1931*

The fruits were an important aboriginal food.

The berries have a special action upon the glands of the reproductive system, as mammae, ovaries, prostate, testes, etc., tending to increase their functional activity.   Lloyd

L. Brook's recipe: Mix one-half each of saw palmetto berries with one-half bull nettle root (*Solanam carolinense*). Make a decoction and take a cupful a day. It invigorates sex glands according to L. Brook.

Sesamum orientale; S. indicum: Sesame or benne
A compound decoction of the seeds with linseed is used as an aphrodisiac in the Philippines.   Quisumbing

Sesame was cultivated since ancient times by the Persians and Egyptians. The seeds are highly esteemed by Arabs and people of the East. They were brought to the West Indies and United States by Negroes of Africa. Slaves of the Southern States parched the seeds over fire, boiled them in broths, made puddings and prepared them in various other ways. They made a demulcent drink by steeping one or two fresh leaves in a pint of cool water. Dried leaves were steeped into hot water. The infusion or drink was used for cholera, infantum, diarrhoea, dysentery, catarrh and infections of the urinary passages.

Sesame oil taken internally in large doses is laxative. In the Orient it is much used as a tonic and as an external application to promote softness of the skin.

Sesame oil is now used in great quantities for making margarine, salad oils and good quality cooking oil.

Shorea robusta: Dammar resin tree
An aromatic oleo-resinous gum exudes from the stem; it is the sal dammar of commerce, and locally known as sal or dhooma; it is aphrodisiac.   As an aphrodisiac the resin is taken every morning in 20 grain doses with a pint of boiled milk; or it is fried with clarified butter and then strained through water, the thick layer, left over after decanting the water, is used.   Dastur

Sida cordifolia
The whole plant contains the alkaloid ephedrine, but the seeds contain much more of the active principle, over .3 percent, than

90

the other parts.   The seeds are considered (in India) to be aphrodisiac.   Dastur

Silphium perfoliatum: Ragged cup, Indian cup-plant

The Indians say Indian cup-plant makes an old man young; the inference from which is, that it is a powerful alterative restorative. It is used in strong tea, the root requiring long steeping to extract the strength.   H. Howard

Sium Sisarum: Skirret

The plant was introduced to England about 1548.   Loureirs believed it originated from China and Cochin-China where he says it is cultivated. *Origin of Cultivated Plants* states other botanists have mentioned Japan and Korea, but in these countries there are species which root is easy to confound particularly with *Sium Ninsi* and *Panax ginseng*.   If species of skirret are "confounded" with ginseng, it is very likely they were also fraudulently substituted for the genuine article.

In one short season, skirret produces a root about the size of a six-year-old mature ginseng. Skirret resembles ginseng in color as well as flavor. Skirret root was popularly regarded in Old Europe as an aphrodisiac. Gerarde wrote in 1636, "The women in Suenia [Sweden], saith Hieronymus Heroldus, prepare the roots hereof for their husbands, and know full well wherefore and why, etc."   A few years later Dr. Tho. Venner added, "They are moderately hot, and somewhat moist; they delight the palat, excite the appetite, and are easily concocted [digested]: they comfort the stomack,   and   give,   though   not   much,   yet   commendable nourishment: they also provoke urine, open obstructions and are withall of a venerous windy faculty. They are good for every age and constitution."

Rhind wrote: "The roots of skirret contain a mucilaginous and saccharine matter, and were at one time much esteemed in cookery."   M. Margraaf, a chemist, obtained one and one-third ounces of pure sugar from a half pound of skirret roots. Bohmer

91

observes, that it may profitably be distilled, and converted into brandy. Skirret is not mentioned as an aphrodisiac in Oriental records researched by this writer.

Smilax chinensis: Sarsaparilla or China root
The rhizome has considerable reputation as an aphrodisiac and tonic in the Orient.   Burkill

China root is used in India to some extent like sarsaparilla as tonic and aphrodisiac in the form of decoction (1 in 10 or 2 ounces in a pint of water, and boiled down and reduced to 5); dose is 1 ounce thrice daily. Boiled in milk, flavored with cardamon and cinnamon, it is used for seminal weakness.

Nadkarni

Solanum melongena: Egg plant, aubergine
In Africa the juice of the plant enters into some love philtres. In South Nigeria the egg plant is symbolic of fertility, and used by barren women.   Dalziel

S. indicum: Indian nightshade
According to Nadkarni the plant is a cordial, an aphrodisiac, an astringent, and a resolvent. Kirtikar and Basu report that the root, taken internally, manifests strongly exciting qualities. Perrot and Hurrier say that the fruit is tonic and laxative.

S. nigrum: Black nightshade
Stuart states that the young shoots are eaten, after boiling, and are considered to be corrective, cooling, and tonic to men (increasing virility) and women (benefiting menstrual disorders.)

Quisumbing

Black nightshade is considered a poisonous plant in the United States; however Parmentier, the French agriculturist (1737-1813), claimed the leaves were eaten like spinach in the West Indies and

France. [Many poisonous plants are made edible after being prepared in a special manner]. Quisumbing wrote that an improved variety is edible in the Philippines and the ripe berries make a delightful jam and excellent pies. Analysis of the cultivated variety grown in the Philippines show that they are an excellent source of calcium and phosphorus and a good source of iron.

Sophora flavescens
The root is a bitter tonic and stomachic, considered by some to be better than true ginseng in China.   *Gardens' Bulletin*

Sophoras are grown for their graceful foliage and attractive flowers. *Sophora tomentosa* is said to have medicinal properties and the seeds of *S. secundiflora* contain sophorine, a poisonous alkaloid.

Spanish fly. (See **Cantharis**)

Sphaeranthus hirtus: East Indian globe thistle
Oil prepared from the root by steeping it in water and then boiling it in sesame oil until all the water is expelled, taken on empty stomach every morning for 41 days in doses of *2 dirhems*, is a valuable aphrodisiac.   Nadkarni

Spondias amara
The fruits are regarded as highly favorable to long life, health and the preservation of a youthful appearance.   Stuart, 1911

Spondias mombin, an American variety, is often grown for its excellent flavored fruits. *Spondias lutea*, known as hog-plum, is a handsome tree that bears fruit generally relished only by hogs.

Stephania abyssinica

In Liberia the leaves, cooked in rice, are used by childless women and are said to be effective; the tender parts of the plant being also wrapped around the loins (Cooper).   Dalziel

Strychnos nux-vomica: Strychnine tree, nux-vomica tree, poison nut

Strychnine is one of the most violent poisons of the plant kingdom. One-half to one grain can produce its horrifying toxic symptoms followed by death. Nux vomica contains two alkaloids, strychnine and brusine. Strychnine, as a drug, has the same utility as nux vomica, but it is more powerful, and is very commonly used in western medicine; it is a very useful cardiac tonic, and in great demand as a general tonic and stimulant; it is also much used for sexual debility, impotence and spermatorrhoea; it is given as a tonic for the nervous and muscular systems. As an aid to digestive functions, it is given in very minute doses, usually not more than 1/8 of a grain.   Dastur

S. ignatii: Ignatius bean

An extract of *Ignatia amara* was the base of a celebrated medicine extensively advertised by a highly respectable and retired quack....In overdoses it is an energetic poison. In suitable medicinal doses, it is tonic to the nerves of motion, restoring the natural power and energy.   Thayer, 1876

Seeds [ignatius bean] contain strychnine 15 percent, brucine .5 percent, and proteids; glucoside loganin is believed to be present. Seeds are utilized in Europe for preparing strychnine which they yield in larger quantity than nux-vomica seeds.   Seeds are therefore to be used with great caution.   A tincture known as Tincutra Ignatia is prepared (1 in 10) and administered in doses of 3 to 20 minims as a nerve tonic.   Nadkarni

Tacca involucrata

In some provinces [of Africa] the tuber is regarded either as aphrodisiac or as a charm to beget children, used only by the ruling classes.   Dalziel

Tapir hoofs

"I noticed also that the hoofs of this tapir, which happened to be a male, were divided, marked, and carefully stowed away, as had been done in the case of the other animal (another tapir). Maite explained that the scraping of the tapir's hoofs possess extraordinary properties, but that particular attention must be paid to sex when administering it. On no account should the scrapings from the hoofs of the male tapir be given to a man, nor should those from the female animal be administered to a woman. All the virtues possessed by this strange medicine is annulled if the important question of sex be disregarded, for which reason the hoofs were marked so as to be able to distinguish between the masculine and feminine species afterwards."   Andre, 1900

Millingen mentions, "camels and dromedaries' flesh was much esteemed, their heels most especially."

Tetragastris balsamifera: Bois Cochon

In Haiti the wood of this tree is steeped several days or a week and used as an aphrodisiac.   For greater strength, leane bandee (*Rhynchosia*) is steeped with the wood. The decoction of bois cochon is used as a diuretic and for kidney stones.

Theobroma cacao: Chocolate

Chocolate, the chief drink of the Aztecs, was brought to the Old World in 1526. Like many other New World products, it was regarded as an aphrodisiac. Davenport wrote, "An immoderate use of chocolate was, in the seventeenth century, considered so powerful an aphrodisiac that Jean Franco Raucher strenuously enforced the necessity of forbidding the monks to drink it, adding that if such an interdiction had been laid upon it at an earlier period, the scandal with which that sacred order had been assailed would have been prevented. It is a singular fact that, fearful of losing their character, or, what perhaps, was dearer to them, their chocolate, the worthy cenobites were so diligent in suppressing Raucher's work that four copies only of it are said to be in existence."

Tinospora cordifolia: Heart-leaved moonseed

All parts of the creeper are used medicinally; it is reputed as one of the most valuable medicinal plants by Ayurvedic and Yunani, practitioners [of India]; the fresh plant is considered to be more effective than the dry plant. From the roots and stem is extracted a starchy pulverulent substance having properties similar to those of arrowroot. It is used as an aphrodisiac.   Dastur

Torilis japonica: Hedge-parsley

Mattthiolus in his Commentaries upon Dioscorides, Lib. 2 attributeth unto it many excellent vertues, to provoke venery and bodily lust, and erection of the part.   Gerarde, 1636

Trapa bispinosa: Water chestnut

In Kashmir the water-nuts form a staple farinaceous food. Fruit or nut or seed contains manganese and starch. Used for general debility and seminal weakness.   Nadkarni

It forms one of the important articles of Native sick dietary. It is used in place of Sago or Tapioca, preference being given to it for its taste and flavor. The Chinese also use the dried fruits as an article of food.   Dye, 1867

Tribulus terrestris: Caltrops

The plant is cooling, diuretic, demulcent, tonic, aphrodisiac, and aperient; the fruit and roots have the same properties. The plant, roots and fruit are usually administered in the form of an

96

infusion or decoction; some boil the fruit and roots with rice; the infusion or decoction is taken in large quantities.   Dastur

Trigonella foenum graecum: Fenugreek
The seeds contain the alkaloid trigonelline; they are demulcent, emmenagogue, aromatic, diuretic, nutritive, tonic, emollient, astringent, carminative and aphrodisiac.   Dastur

Farmers in Germany, Hungary and Austria make a decoction of fenugreek seeds and flavor it with mint or lemon and drink it as an aphrodisiac. Fenugreek is one of man's oldest medicinals. Fenugreek seeds are a rich source of protein, vitamins, minerals and trace elements. The ground seeds are used to fatten animals for livestock shows. A noted botanist and agricultural explorer wrote, "Fenugreek boiled with milk and honey was used in Tunis to fatten women for the marriage market." The botanist saw women weighing over 300 pounds!

Truffles. (See Tuber)

Tuber melanosporum, T. aestivum, T. brumale: Truffles
Truffles are underground fruit of the above species of fungi. They are hunted by smell, by pigs or trained dogs. The latter is preferred because pigs often eat the truffles before they can be retrieved. The erotic properties of truffles and mushrooms are considered by most writers as better established than those of fish. The ancient Romans were well acquainted with truffles, and obtained them from Greece and Africa, especially from the province of Libya, the fungi found there being particularly esteemed for their delicacy and flavor. In modern times, also, the truffle is regarded as the "diamond" of the kitchen, being highly valued for its capability of exciting the genesiac sense, it being a positive aphrodisiac which disposes men to be exacting and women complying.   Davenport, 1869

97

Turnera diffusa var. aphrodisiaca: Damiana

Although the physiological action of this plant is only partly known, it is noted that it produces abundant urination and will increase sexual power. It is believed to act on the spinal cord, and some physicians have used it as a brain tonic and a tonic to increase genital function. It has been scientifically accepted as producing favorable reactions in diseases resulting from weakness of the nervous system. Since times immemorial, the Indians, especially in northern Mexico, have been using this plant for muscular and nervous weakness by drinking the mashed leaves as tea. It is also used as an aphrodisiac, and from 1874 to the present time it has been considered by the United States as an excellent tonic. It is also used for catarrhal inflammation of the bladder, and for deficient function of the sexual organs, especially in cases of sexual impotence caused by excesses. It has been used for spermatorrhea, and for orchitis resulting in atrophy of the testicles. It has been used in nephritis amaurosis caused by the excessive use of tobacco.   Martinez

The drug has been almost eulogized for its positive aphrodisiac effects, acting energetically upon the genito-urinary organs of both sexes, removing impotence in the one, and frigidity in the other, whether due to abuses or age. Many physicians who have tried it, deny its possession of such virtues, but friends of the drug attribute their failures to use of the spurious articles.

Felter and Lloyd, 1898

Turnip. (See Brassica rapa)

Urtica dioica: Nettle or stinging nettle

The same [nettle seed] dronken with sweete wine, doth stirre up bodily pleasure, and is good against the blasting and windinesse of the stomacke.   Dodoens, 1586

98

The seed of Nettle stirreth up lust, especially drunke with Cute. Gerarde, 1636

The Seed [of nettle] provokes Venery, if the fresh Seed be boiled, and eaten with Butter for three Days; or eat Hasle [hazel] Nut-Kernels, preserved with Honey; or drink Birch Water, or Wine; or foment the Genitals with a Decoction of Columbine Seed and Herb. Stockerus wrote the Powder of Nettle-seed given in warm Wine, from half a Dram to a Dram, or of Rocket-seed excite Venery. An ointment with Oil or Powder of Ants Eggs, rubbed on the Testicles, is also good; or Stinging the Part with fresh Nettles. Short, 1746

Scottish legend:
"If they wad drink Nettles in March
And at Muggins (Mugwort) in May,
Sae mony braw maidens
Wad not go to clay."

The seeds taken inwardly in moderate quantity excite the system, especially *les plaisirs de l'amour*, and are very forcing, therefore should be cautiously employed. Twenty or thirty grains produce vomiting. Excessive corpulency may be reduced by taking a few of these seeds daily. Thornton, 1814

Stinging nettle herb contains preponderate amounts of organic constituents.

Vanilla plainfolia: Vanilla
Vanilla is an orchid: the royal family of the vegetable kingdom. Its high place in the culinary world more than compensates for its lack of showy flowers. Vanilla is perhaps the most popular of all flavors and has long been regarded as an aphrodisiac. If this were true, we may attribute the population explosion to this most delicate orchid. Genuine vanilla adds a

flavor and fragrant royal elegance to almost any use it is put to. It was a popular ingredient of many love philters and seductive perfumes. Genuine vanilla should not be confused with synthetic imitation vanillin. The difference is far greater than the name similarity.

Verbascum thapsus: Mullein
Seeds considered aphrodisiac in India.   Nadkarni

Mullein leaves and flowers, as well as the root, were much used in folk medicine in Europe and America.

Vernonia amygdalina: Bitter Leaf
The leaves are sold in African markets; the bitterness is diminished by boiling, or the young leaves are soaked in several changes of water and used in soup; they are antiscorbutic and a digestive tonic. A form of the special food is made from the leaves along with butter, condiments, etc.; this may be taken by men merely as a food, but by women in the belief that it renders them sexually more attractive.   Dalziel

Veronica officinalis: Common speedwell
An infusion of the leaves, drank constantly in the manner of tea, is a strengthener, and provocative to venery; and is, by some, ridiculously supposed to be a cure for barrenness.   Green, 1820

A modern German source states that the herb stimulates glandular action and is a blood purifier.

The plant was formerly very extensively used both in Sweden and Germany, as a substitute for tea, and it had the old French name of The de l'Europe.... Speedwell tea was believed by our fathers not only to afford present refreshment, but also to strengthen the frame.   Pratt, 1855

Vinca major: Periwinkle

Periwinkle was of old considered to be a potent aphrodisiac. In *The Boke of Albertus Magnus* we find: "Perwynke when it is beate unto powder with worms of ye earth wrapped about it and with an erbe called houslyke [*Sempervivum tectorum*], it induceth love between man and wyfe if it bee used in their meales."

Macleod

V. rosea: Periwinkle, little pinkie, bright eyes

This species was much used in folk practice whenever the plant was found. A brew of the herb was used by gypsies for diabetes. In Haiti the writer was informed an infusion of the flowers "will lower sugar in the system." Potter lists the herb as astringent, tonic and reputed to be useful in menorrhagia and haemorrhages generally.

In the early 1960s an alkaloid derived from *Vinca rosea* was hailed as a promising drug in the early treatment against a variety of malignancies, including leukemia and Hodgkin's disease.

Waltheria americana

This herb or shrub is mentioned in records over much of the tropical world and said to have a variety of medicinal uses in different regions. Perhaps the most conflicting use comes from Africa. In the gold Coast it is used to cause abortion and in South Africa it is used as a remedy for sterility.   Dalziel

Watercress. (See Nasturtium officinale)

Wine

It restoreth strength most of all other things, and that speedily: It maketh a man merry and joyful: It putteth away feare, care, troubles of minde, and sorrow: It moveth pleasure and lust of the body, and bringeth sleepe gently. . . .

Almighty God for the comfort of mankinde ordained Wine; but decreed withall, that it should be moderately taken, for so it is wholsome and comfortable: but when measure is turned into excesse, it becommeth unwholesome, and a poyson most venomous, relaxing the sinews, bringing with it the palsy and falling sickness: to those of a middle age it bringeth hot fevers, frensie, and lecherie; it consumeth the liver and other of the inward parts: besides, how little credence is to be given to drunkards it is evident; for though they be mighty men, yet it maketh them monsters, and worse than brute beasts. Finally in a word to conclude; this excessive drinking of Wine dishonoreth Noblemen, beggereth the poore, and more have beene destroied by surfeiting therewith, than by the sword.

Gerarde, 1636

Withania somnifera: Winter cherry

The root contains the alkaloid sominferine. It is a powerful tonic, stimulant, alterative, aphrodisiac, narcotic, diuretic, and deobstruent; in indigenous medicine it is given in 30 grain doses, in general debility. Half to one drachm of the powdered root with milk or clarified butter is used as an aphrodisiac and in seminal debility. Dastur

Powder of the root mixed with ghee and honey in equal parts is recommended for impotence or seminal debility; it is to be taken in the evening, followed by milk. As a nutrient and health restorative to the pregnant and old people a decoction of the root is recommended; or its powder with milk may be taken. The decoction boiled down with milk and with ghee added to the mixture is recommended for curing the sterility of women. It is to be taken for a few days, soon after the menstrual period.

Nadkarni

Wrightia tinctoria: Sweet indrajao

Seeds are sweet and tonic, and are given (in India) for seminal weakness. Nadkarni

Xylopia aethiopica: African, Guinea or Ethiopian pepper. Spice tree

The decoction of the fruit or bark, or both used as medicine. As a women's remedy it is taken to encourage fertility and in childbed.   Dalziel

Yohimbe. (See **Pansinystalia yohimba**)

Zanthoxylum rhetsa

Native of India and occasionally cultivated in Ceylon. Fruit is useful as a condiment in curries. Bark is aphrodisiac and bitter aromatic.   Nadkarni

Zingiber officinale: Ginger, Jamaica ginger

In Senegal and French Guinea, ginger is said to be chewed after kola nut, the effect being to enhance the properties of the latter, and being regarded as itself aphrodisiac, the two are correspondingly more stimulating.   Dalziel

Kola nuts have a high caffeine content. Ginger is more efficacious as a tea when your have lost count on cocktails; good for grandma and grandpa as a stomach warmer; for teenage girls as an occasional tea; good for Johnny after eating green apples and when colds threaten.   Little need be added to ginger's many culinary and beverage uses.

ANAPHRODISIACS

Agents which diminish the sexual appetite and lower its functional power, either by depressing the special nervous apparatus or by decreasing the local circulation.

Albizzia lebbeck: Woman's tongue, shack-shack
Sanyal and Ghose report that the flowers possess the power of causing retention of the seminal fluid.   Quisumbing

The tree is quite pretty when in full bloom and quite ugly when it sheds its leaves and the dry pods rattle incessantly in the wind, whence several of its common names. The chief value of the tree is for its wood, which is hard, heavy and takes a good finish.

Alcoholic beverages
Even the ancients recognized the debilitating effects of intoxicating compounds on the reproductive functions. "Venus drowned in Bacchus" was one of their proverbial expressions; and who is not familiar with the philosophical disquisition on drinking and lechery, which the porter in Macbeth reads to Macdufff: "Lechery, sir, drinking provokes and unprovokes: it provokes the desire but it takes away the performance; it makes him and it mars him; it sets him on, and it takes him off; it persuades him, and it disheartens him."   Napheys, 1871

Napheys also added, "Drunkards and tipplers suffer early loss of virility."

107

Anethum graveolens: Dill
Such as have a dim Sight, and are sluggish to Venery, should refrain [from] this herb.   Short, 1746

Angelica archangelica: Angelica
The dried root of Angelica made into powder, and taken in wine or other drinke, will abate the rage of lust in young persons, as I have it related unto me upon credit.   Parkinson, 1629

Women of ancient China wore angelica seeds with other fragrant drugs in their girdles.   The seeds were specially considered to be a woman's drug.

Artemisia absinthium: Wormwood
The use of the Herb checks immoderate Venery.   Short, 1746

The doctor probably meant excessive use.   (See **Artemisia absinthium** in **Aphrodisiacs.**)

Camphor. (See **Cinnamomum camphora**)

Carica papaya: Papaya, pawpaw
In Jamaica, medicine men believe the milk from the stalk is detrimental to male virility.

Cicuta maculata, C. maculatum and other Cicuta species: Poison hemlock
Hemlocke is verie evill, dangerous, hurtfull, and venemous, in so much that whosoever taketh of it, dieth, except he drink good old wine after it: for the drinking of such wine, after the receiving of Hemlocke togither, the strength of the poison is augmented, and then it killeth out of hand, insomuch he is no kinde of waies to be holpen, that hath taken Hemlocke with wine.   Dodoens, 1586

Hemlock being a Poison, is not used inwardly, but outwardly. A Poultise of the Leaves, laid to the Cods, extinguishes Lust strongly; there it is neither applied in Poultises alone to that Part in Man, nor to Women's Breasts in Inflammations; but it is usefully and safely laid to any other inflamed Part of the Body; it repels the Heat from creeping Ulcers, occasioned by sharp Humours.
                                                        Short, 1746

Lust to abate, stampe it [hemlock], and apply it to the pecten.
                                                    Langham, 1633

It is said a small piece of poison hemlock taken internally has been known to cause fatal poisoning.

Cinnamomum camphora: Camphor
The ancients had a high opinion of camphor, a reputation which this drug preserved until, comparatively, a late period, for Scaliger informs that, in the seventeenth century, monks were compelled to smell and masticate it for the purpose of extinguishing concupiscence; and it was a favorite maxim of the medical school of Salernum that: "Camphor if smell'd; A man will geld."

This fatal property, however, has been denied by modern medical authorities, and apparently with reason, if the fact be true that such workmen as are employed in extracting this useful vegetable product, and who may be said to live constantly in a highly camphorated atmosphere, do not find themselves in the least degree incapacitated for gratifying the calls of l'amour physique.
                                                        Davenport

Burton asserts the value of camphor as an anti-aphrodisiac, and says that when fastened to the parts of generation, or carried in the breeches, it renders the virile member flaccid.

Coffea arabica: Coffee

In the year 1695 it was maintained, in a thesis at the Ecole de Medicine at Paris, that the daily use of coffee deprived both man and woman of the generative powers. Abernethy, the celebrated surgeon, said: "Any man that drinks coffee and soda water, and smokes cigars, may lie with my wife."   Davenport

Coffee in moderation has rather a tonic than an enervating effect; but in excess, it is distinctly proven by repeated instances that it quite prostrates the sexual faculties.   Napheys, 1871

Cucumis melo: Musk melon

It is harder of digestion than is any of the Cucumbers, and if it remaine long in the stomack it putrifieth, and is occasion of pestilent fevers. Which thing also Aetius witnesseth, in the first booke of *Tetrabibles;* writing the use of Cucumeres or Cucumbers breedeth pestilent fevers: for hee also taketh Cucumis to be that which is commonly called a Melon; which is usually eaten of the Italians and Spaniards rather to represse the rage of lust, than for any other physicall vertue. The seed is of like operation with that of the former Cuccumber.   Gerarde, 1636

Erythroxylon coca or E. truxillense: Cocaine

A drop of a 4 percent solution of Cocaine upon the glans penis will destroy all erection-power for a quarter to half an hour.

Potter

Hieracium species; Hawkweeds

It softly invites Sleep, checks Venery, and Venereal Dreams.
Short, 1746

Hawkweeds may have mild narcotic properties similar to its related species Lactuca.

110

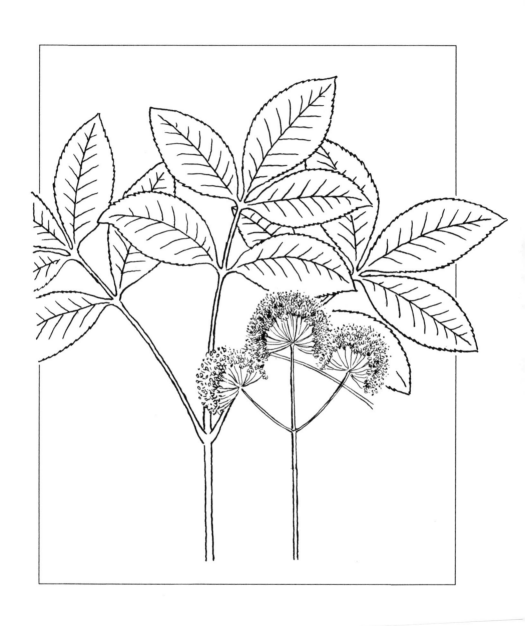

AMERICAN SARSAPARILLA
(*v. Smilax*)
See page 92

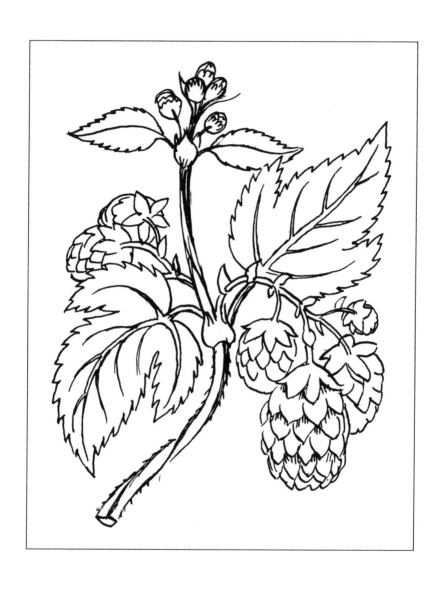

HOPS
(*Humulus lupulus*)
See page 111

Humulus lupulus: Hops

The Lupulin is a powerful anaphrodisiac, composer of the genital organs and quieter of painful erections. In a large number of cases of painful erections, dependent upon gonorrhea, lupulin quieted the erethisms, in four-fifths.

Tilden, 1858

Hops have a tendency to produce sleep. A pillow stuffed with hop strobiles is also useful in allaying restlessness and producing sleep in nervous disorders. Hops are used in great quantities in the manufacture of beer.

Lactuca sativa: Lettuce

Lettuce leaves probably possess, in a very mild degree, soporific properties. The ancients considered them antiaphrodisiac. The flowering plant is more powerful and produces, in a feeble degree, the effects of lacturacium. Lettuce also possesses slight hypnotic properties. It may be taken with advantage at supper to promote sleep. (Lactucarium, or lettuce opium, mentioned in the old pharmacopoeias, is the concrete, milky juice of the plant). It is supposed that the seeds, by relaxing the genital organs, diminish the spermatic secretion.

Quisumbing

Mentha spicata: Spearmint

It eases Children Gripes, strengthens the Brain and Memory, and checks immoderate Venereal Desires.   Short, 1746

(See **Mentha** in **Aphrodisiacs.**)

Nicotiana tabacum: Tabacco

Physicians who have the opportunity of watching operatives in tobacco-factories, have reported that the males frequently suffer from sexual debility.   Napheys, 1871

111

Nitre: Saltpeter

A man, by profession a musician, of an athletic figure and sanguine complexion, with red hair, and a very warm temperament, was so tormented with erotic desires that the venereal act, repeated several times in the course of a few hours, failed to satisfy him. Disgusted with himself, and fearing, as a religious man, the punishment with which concupiscense is threatened in the Gospel, he applied to a medical practitioner, who prescribed bleeding and the use of sedatives and refrigerants, together with a light diet.   Having found no relief from this course of treatment, he was then recommended to have recourse to wedlock, and, in consequence, married a robust and healthy young woman, the daughter of a farmer. At first, the change appeared to benefit him, but, in a short time, he tired his wife out by his excessive lubricity, and relapsed into his former satyriasis. His medical friend now recommended frequent fasting, together with prayer, but these also failing of effect, the unhappy man proposed to submit to castration, an operation which was judged to be highly improper considering the great risk the patient must necessarily incur. The latter, however, still persisted that his wish should be complied with, when, fortunately, a case having occurred in Paris, in which a person afflicted with nephritic pains occasioned by the presence of a calculus, was cured by a preparation of nitre, at the expense,   however, of being forever incapacitated for the pleasures of love, the hint was taken, and doses of nitre dissolved in *aqua nymphea* were given, night and morning,   during the space of eight days and with such success that, at the end of that time,   he could scarcely satisfy the moderate claims of his wife.   Davenport, 1869

Nymphaea alba

The roote and seed of the white water Lillie are very good against Venus, or fleshly desires, if one drinke the decoction thereof, or use the pouder of the sayd seed and roote in meates

112

[food]: for it drieth up the seed of generation, and so causeth to live in chastitie. The same propertie is in the roote, as Plinie writeth, if it be brused and applied outwardly to the secret parts.

Dodoens, 1586

The root and seed of great water Lilly is very good against venerie or fleshly desire, if one drink the decoction of it, or use the seed or root in pouder in his meats: for it drieth up the seed of generation, and so causeth a man to be chaste, especially used in broth with flesh.

Gerarde, 1636

Nymphaea: White water-lily
Nelumbo lutea: Yellow water-lily

There is the white and black, the first hath a yellow Flower, and white Root; the last a white Flower, and black Root; both of them [when] dry, bind and cleanse. The former dries most, the latter cleanses most. It dries without Biting of Sharpness, therefore the Ancients used it not only in Loosenesses and Bloody Fluxes, but for the Whites. The Roots and Seeds of the White Lilly (which is mostly used when it can be got, but, in Want of it, the other may be taken) cool, dry, and bind. The Leaves and Flowers cool and moisten; both of them are of great Benefit in Fluxes of the Belly; but especially seminal, nocturnal Pollutions [emissions], whether voluntary or involuntary; whether from the Heat, Sharpness, or Thinness of the Seed of Blood: So very powerful are they in subduing Lust, beyond any, or all other *British* Plants, says Prosper Alpinus, that Monks, Nuns, Friars, and Hermits, that would live chastely, drink daily, for twelve Days together, a Dram of it, and Syrup of poppies; this, Inclination, and Power of Coition; therefore do the Aegyptions dread and avoid it. In a Priapism, Galen always gave a little of it with Success. And Avicenna cried out how it lessens Pollution, and quite erases Venereal Desire; nay, even frequent Anointing the Genitals with it, or the Stomach, Reins, or Bladder, it will produce the same Effect; and is therefore much better than a

Poultise of bruised Hemlock laid to the Testicles, which only abates the Fury of Lust for a few Hours.   Short, 1746

Some physicians place great confidence in the medicines called refrigerants.   The most favorite of these are infusions from the leaves or the flowers of the white water-lily. According to Pliny, the white water-lily was considered so powerful that those who take it for twelve days successively will then find themselves incapable of propagating their species, and if it be used for forty days, the amorous propensity will be entirely extinguished.
                                                        Davenport, 1869

Origanum majorana: Marjoram

The following was taken from a treatise on Sexual Passion by Dr. Gallavardin of Lyons, France, written in the late 1800s: The person who discovered a remedy that, in a certain sense may be considered as a specific against sexual passion, was a clergyman of Mizza, the founder of an orphan asylum.   This remedy is *Origanum majorana*, which proves effective in masturbation and in excessively aroused sexual impulses. The author uses it in the 4th dilution, as he has not found the higher potencies effective. He dissolves 5 or 6 globules of this dilution in 4 teaspoonfuls of fresh water, and the young masturbator takes of this every 2 days, a quarter of an hour before the meal, 1 teaspoonful. If the cure is not accomplished 8 days after this solution is used up, the same dose is repeated in the same way.   When desired, this remedy can be used,   according to the author, without the knowledge of the patient, by pouring a teaspoonful into the soup, milk or chocolate. The effect frequently appears very rapidly, but sometimes it does not appear.   Anshutz

Portulaca oleracea: Purslane

They use to eate the garden and Wilde Purcelaine in Salades and Meates as they do Lettuce, but it cooleth the blood, and maketh it waterie, and nourisheth verie little, yet for all that it is

114

good for those that have great heat in their stomackes and inwarde parts.   Dodoens, 1586

The same taken in like manner is good for the bladder and kidnies, and allaieth the outragious lust of the body: the juyce also hath the same vertue.   Gerarde, 1636

It checks Lust, hinders Venereal Dreams, and nocturnal Pollutions, therefore good for the Lovers of Chastity, and the too Lascivious.   Short, 1746

Potassium bromide

Doctor W.J. Robinson records the following: Some high-minded young men, considering extramarital intercourse morally wrong, decided to repress their sexual desires by the use of potassium bromide. At the advice of a young physician they took 30 to 60 grains (2 to 4 grams) every night for a period of several months. Two of the young men kept up the bromide, with some intermissions, for over two years. Most of them succeeded in repressing and in suppressing their desires. But, unfortunately, they also succeeded in several other things: they succeeded in ruining their digestion, in getting a nice crop of bromide-acne that was very resistant to treatment, and in becoming impotent.

Potassium bromide is used as a nerve sedative, and antispasmodic.

Ruta graveolens: Rue, Herb of Grace

The School of Salernum was the earliest medical educational center in Christian Europe founded about 800 A.D. For the sake of clarity, simplicity and brevity the principles of the school were reduced to poems. A physician who could not quote the poems was looked upon with suspicion. The following was taken from John Ordronaux's translation of *Code of Health of the School of Salernum*, 1870:

Of use to sight, a noble plant is Rue;

115

O blear-eyed man, 'twill sharpen sight for you!
In men, it curbs love's strongest appetite,
In women, tends to amplify its might.
Let rue to chastity inclines mankind,
Gives power to see and sharpens, too, the mind;
And instantly, when in decoction, frees
Your house for-ever from tormenting fleas.

Rue eaten in meate, or otherwise used by a certaine space of time, quencheth and drieth up nature, and naturall seede of man, and the milke in the breasts of women that give sucke.

Dodoens, 1586

Rue eaten greens, quencheth lust in men, and provoketh lust in women, and sharpeneth the sight and wit.   Langham, 1633

It is a great Preserver of Chastity.   Short, 1746

Rosa species: Rose
Their Leaves (petals) laid under the Back at Night check Lust and diminish Seed.   Short, 1746

The above does not conform with Nadkarni. (See **Rosa** in **Aphrodisiacs.**)

Salix alba: Willow
The desire for coition was supposed to be diminished by drinking a decoction of the pounded leaves of willow.

Davenport, 1869

Willow was used for ages in folk practice as fomentation for pains of almost any kind. In 1827 a French chemist isolated salicin from willow; however the chemical could not be taken internally. In 1838 salicylic acid was made from salicin and in 1899 a German chemist made acetylsalicyle acid which finally

116

could be taken internally for the relief of pains. This product now is best known as aspirin.

In 1971 two researchers of the Royal College of Surgeons (England) reported that aspirin taken in ordinary doses may affect men's fertility. It is remarkable how many folk practices prove sound.

S. nigra: Willow catkins

In cases of excessive venereal desire, amounting to satyriasis, from experience I would use this remedy first. I have seen it control the venereal appetite in a very satisfactory manner. It can be given in cases where the bromides have always been considered appropriate, and it can be given where the bromides would be very inappropriate and there is no reflex effect on the brain or nervous system. The fresh catkins of willow are macerated in twice their weight of alcohol.　　　　Anshutz

Saltpeter or Saltpetre. (See Nitre)

Vegetable diet

From ancient times it has been well known that a wholly or chiefly vegetable diet favors the subjugation of the passions, and hence it was recommended to persons of violent desires, and enjoined on celibate orders of priesthood. Particularly those vegetables which contain a large percentage of vegetable fibre and of water, as cabbage, turnips, beets, melons, and carrots, and those which contain acids and some soporific principle, as sorrel, sour fruits, lettuce, endive, and other salads, are reported to have especial virtues in this direction.　　　　Napheys, 1871

BIBLIOGRAPHY

Anon. *The Family Companion for Health, or Plain, Easy and Certain Rules which being punctually observed and followed, will keep Families from diseases and procure Them a Long Life.* London, 1730.

Anshutz, E.P. *New, Old and Forgotten Remedies.* Philadelphia, 1900.

Aurand, Samuel H. *Botanical Materia Medica and Pharmacology.* 1899.

Bailey, L.H. *The Standard Cyclopedia of Horticulture.* New York, 1933.

Bayley, Iris. "The Bush-Teas of Barbados" in *The Journal of the Barbados Museum and Historical Society*, Vol. XVI, No. 3, May 1949.

Bell, Hesketh J. *Obeah: Witchcraft in the West Indies.* London, 1893.

Berdoe, Edward. *The Origin and Growth of the Healing Art.* London, 1893.

Bingley, Rev. William. *Useful Knowledge or A Familiar and Explanatory Account of the Various Productions of Nature, Mineral, Vegetable and Animal.* London, 1816.

Brutus, Timolen, C. and A.V. Pierre-Noel. *Les Plantes et Le Legumes D'Haiti Qui Guerissent.* Tome II. Port-Au-Prince, Haiti, 1960.

Burkill, I.H. *A Dictionary of the Economic Products of the Malay Peninsula.* Published on Behalf of the Governments of the Straits Settlements and Federated Malay States by the Crown Agents for the Colonies. London, 1935.

Caius, J.F. "The Medicinal and Poisonous Spurges of India" in *The Journal of The Bombay Natural History Society*, No. 40, 1940.

Carles, W.R. *Life in Corea.* London and New York, 1888.

Clarke, John H. *A Dictionary of Practical Materia Medica.* Edinburgh, 1962.

Collymore, Frank A. *Notes For A Glossary Of Words And Phrases Of Barbadian Dialect.* Bridgetown, Barbados, 1957. *Contributions from the United States National Herbarium.* Vol. 23, part 3. Washington, 1923

Cook, O.F, and G.N. Collins. *Economic Plants of Puerto Rico.* Washington, 1903.

Covey, A. Dale. *The Secrets of Specialists.* Newark, 1911.

Coxe, John Redman. *The American Dispensatory, Containing the Operations of Pharmacy, Together With the Natural, Chemical, Pharmaceutical and Medical History of the Different Substances Employed in Medicine.* 4th ed. Philadelphia, 1818.

Dalziel, J.M. *The Useful Plants of West Tropical Africa. Published on behalf of the Federal Government of Nigeria, and the Governments of the Gold Coast, Sierra Leone and Gambia.* London, 1955.

Dastur, J.F. *Medicinal Plants of India and Pakistan.* Bombay, 1962.

Davenport, J. *Aphrodisiacs and Anti-aphrodisiacs: Three Essays on the Power of Reproduction; With Some Account Of The Judicial "Congress" As Practiced In France During The Seventeenth Century.* London, 1869.

Dey, Kenny Loll. *The Indigenous Drugs of India; or Short Descriptive Notices of the Medicines, Both Vegetable and Mineral, in Common Use Among the Natives of India.* 1867.

Dodoens, D. Rembert. *A New Herball, or History Of Plants: Wherein is contained the whole discourse and perfect description of all sorts of Herbes and Plants: Their divers and sundrie kindes: and that not onely of those which are heere growing in this our Countrie of England, but of all others also of forraine Realms commonly used in Physicke First set foorth in the Douch or Almaigne toong, by that learned D. Rembert Dodoens, Physition to the Emperor: And now first translated*

120

out of French into English, by Henrie Lyte, esquier. London, 1586.

Drury, C.H. *The useful Plants of India.* 1873.

Dymock, W. *The Vegetable Materia Medica of Western India.* 1885.

Felter, Harvey Wickes and John Uri Lloyd. *King's American Dispensatory.* 1898.

Gerarde, John. *The Herball or Generall Historie of Plantes.* Gathered by John Gerarde of London in Chivrgerie. Very much Enlarged and Amended by Thomas Johnson Citizen and Apothecarye of London. London, 1636.

Green, Thomas. *The Universal Herbal, or Botanical Medical and Agricultural Dictionary.* Liverpool, 1820.

Guerrero, L.M. *Medicinal Uses of Philippine Plants.* Manila, 1921.

Guilfoyle, W.R. *Australian Botany.* 1884.

Gumpel, C. Godfrey. *Common Salt. Its Use and Necessity for the Maintenance of Health and the Prevention of Disease.* London, 1898.

Hand, Wm. M. *The House Surgeon and Physician; designed to Assist Heads of Families, Travellers, and Sea-faring People, in Discerning, Distinguishing, and Curing Diseases; with Concise Directions for the Preparation and use of a numerous collection of The Best American Remedies: together with Many of the most approved, from the shop of the Apothecary. All in Plain English.* New-Haven, 1820.

Hocking, George M. *A Dictionary of Terms in Pharmacognosy.* Springfield, Illinois, 1955.

Hooper, D. "On Chinese Medicine: Drugs of Chinese Pharmacies in Malay" in *Gardens Bulletin Straits Settlements.* Vol. VI, 1929.

Howard, Horton. *An Improved System of Botanic Medicine.* Cincinnati, 1854.

Howard, Richard A. *The Vegetation of the Grenadines, Windward Islands, British West Indies.* Cambridge, 1952.

Kolbl's Krauterfibel. Munchen, 1972.

Lahontan, Baron De. *New Voyages to North-America. Reprinted from the English edition of 1703.* Chicago, 1905.

Langham, William. *The Garden of Health; Containing the sundry rare and hidden vertues and properties of all kindes of Simples and Plants.* London, 1633.

Leyel, Mrs. C.F. *The Magic of Herbs.* London, 1926.

Li, H.L. *The Garden Flowers of China.* New York, 1959.

Lindley, John. *Flora Medica; A Botanical account of all the more important Plants Used in Medicine in Different parts of the World.* London, 1838.

Macleod, Dawn. *A Book of Herbs.* London, 1968.

Martinez, Maximo. *Medicinal Herbs of Mexico.* Mexico, D.F., 1933.

Miller, Joseph. *Botanicum Officinale; Or a Compendious Herbal: Giving an Account of all Plants as are now used in the Practice of Physick.* London, 1722.

Miller, Philip. *The Gardeners Dictionary: Containing the Methods of Cultivating and Improving The Kitchen, Fruit and Flower Garden, As Also The Physick Garden, Wilderness, Conservatory and Vineyard; According to the Practice of the Most Experienced Gardeners of the Present Age.* London, 1737.

Millingen, J.G. *Curiosities of Medical Experience.* London, 1839.

Millspaugh, Charles F. *American Medical Plants.* Philadelphia, 1887.

Monroe, John. *The American Botanist and Family Physician.* 1824.

Nadkarni, K.M. *Indian Materia Medica.* Third ed. Bombay, [n.d.]

Napheys, George H. *The Transmission of Life.* Philadelphia, 1871.

Nehrling, Henry. *My Garden in Florida.* Estero, Florida, 1944.

Nickell, J.M. *Botanical Ready Reference.* Chicago, 1911.

Ochse, J.J. *Vegetables of the Dutch East Indies.* 1931.

Paris, J.A. *Pharmacologia.* London, 1833.

Parkinson, John. *Paradisi In Sole / Paradisus Terrestris. Faithfully reprinted from the edition of 1629.* London, 1904.

Parkinson. *Theatrum Botanicum: The Theater of Plants Or, An Herball Of A Large Extent: Containing therein a more ample and exact History and declaration of the Physicall Herbs and plants that are in other Authors, encreased by the accesse of many hundreds of new rare, and strange Plants from all the parts of the world, with sundry Gummes, and other Physicall materials, than hath beene hitherto published by any before; And a most large demonstration of their Natures and Vertues.* London, 1640.

Pechey, J. *A Plain Introduction To The Art of Physick. Containing The Fundamentals, And Necessary Preliminaries to Practice.* London, 1697.

Phillips, Henry. *The Companion For The Kitchen Garden.* London, 1831.

Potter, O.L. *Quiz-Compends-Materia Medica.* London, 1911.

Pratt, Anne. *The Flowering Plants, Grasses, Sedges & Ferns of Great Britain.* Edinburgh, 1855.

Quisumbing, Eduardo. *Medicinal Plants of the Philippines.* Manila, 1951.

Rhind, William. *A History of the Vegetable Kingdom.* London, 1868.

Robinson, J. *A Practical Treatise On The Causes, Symptoms, And Treatment of Sexual Impotence And Other Sexual Disorders In Men And Women.* New York, 1915.

Rogler, Gustl. *Krauterwunder.* Munich, 1949.

Safford, William Edwin. *The Useful Plants of the Island of Guam.* Washington, 1905.

Salmon, William. *The Family Dictionary or Household Companion.* London, 1710.

Sanyal, D. and R. Ghose. *Vegetable drugs of India.* 1934.

Short, Tho. *Medicina Britannica Or, A Treatise on Such Physical Plants, As Are Generally to be found in the Fields or Gardens*

123

in Great-Britain Containing a particular Account of their Nature, Virtues, and Uses. London, 1746.

Smith, John. A Dictionary of Popular Names of the Plants which furnish the Natural and Acquired Wants of Man, in all matters of Domestic and General Economy: Their History, Products and Uses. London, 1882.

Standley, Paul C. Trees and Schrubs of Mexico. Washington, 1920.

Stuart, Rev. G.A. Chinese Materia Medica. Extensively revised from Dr. F. Porter Smith's work. Shanghai, 1911.

Sturrock, David. Tropical Fruits for Southern Florida and Cuba and Their Uses. Gainesville, Fla., 1940.

Thayer, Henry. Descriptive Catalogue of Fluid and Solid Extracts in Vacus, also Concentrations and Officinal Pills Prepared by Henry Thayer and Company. Cambridgeport, Mass., 1876.

Thorton, John Robert. A Family Herbal: or Familiar Account of The Medical Properties of British and Foreign Plants. London, 1814.

Tilden and Company. Formulae for making Tinctures, Infusions, Syrups, Wines, Mixtures, Pills, etc., Simple and Compound, from the Fluid & Solid Extracts, prepared at the Laboratory of Tilden & Co. New Lebanon, N.Y., [n.d.]

Uphof, J.C. Th. Dictionary of Economical Plants. Weinsheim, Germany, 1959.
The Useful and Ornamental Plants in Trinidad and Tobago. Port-of-Spain Trinidad, 1951.

Venner, Tho. Via Recta Ad Vitam Longam, Or A treatise wherein the right way and best manner of living for attaining to a long and healthfull life, is clearly demonstrated and punctually applied to very age and constitution of the body. London, 1650.

Voisin, Andre. Soil, Grass and Cancer. London, 1959.

Whitlaw, Charles. Whitlaw's New Medical Discoveries, with A Defence of the Linnaean Doctrine, and a translation of his

Vegetable Materia Medica, which now first appears in an English Dress. London, 1829.

Williams, R.O. *The Useful and Ornamental Plants of Zanzibar and Pemba.* Zanzibar, 1949.

Willich, A.F.M. *The Domestic Encyclopaedia, or a dictionary of facts and useful knowledge.* London, 1802.

Wren, R.C. *Potter's Cyclopaedia of Botanical Drugs and Preparations.* London, 1932.

COMMON AND LATIN NAMES OF PLANTS

Plants in this book are listed alphabetically by their Latin names as common names are frequently confusing and often refer to unrelated species.

Readers more familiar with common plant names should read this list to find the common plant names they are seeking. Then note the equivalent Latin names and refer to the Latin names in the text.

Many of the plants mentioned in this book are considered weeds in their native countries or are only grown locally in gardens and are not marketed. However, plants which can often be found in grocery or ethnic food stores are noted by an asterik (*). Plants which can often be found in herb, health food or drug stores are noted by a cross (+).

Abyssinian tea	Catha edulis
African pepper	Xylopia aethiopica
American Ginseng+	Panax quinquefolia
American mandrake+	Podophyllum peltatum
Anatto*	Bixa orellana
Angelica+	Angelica archangelica
Anise/Aniseed+	Pimpinella anisum
Arabian manna	Alhagi maurorum
Arnatto (Anatto)*	Bixa orellana
Artichoke*	Cynara scolymus
Ash tree	Fraxinus excelsior
Asparagus*	Asparagus officinalis
Aubergine (Egg plant)*	Solanum melongena
Avocado*	Persea americana
Babul	Acacia arabica
Baldmony	Meum athamanticum
Balsam-pear	Momordica balsamina
Barrenwort	Epimedium sagittatum

Bauhinia pods	Bauhinia esculenta
Bawdwort	Meum athamanticum
Bead tree	Adenanthera pavonina
Benne (Sesame seed)+	Sesamum orientale, S. indicum
Betel pepper	Piper betle
Bimlipitum jute	Hibiscus cannabinus
Bitter leaf	Vernonia amygdalina
Black nightshade	Solanum nigrum
Blister beetle	Cantharis vesicatoria
Bloodveined sage	Salvia haematodes
Bois Bande	Hieronyma caribaea
Bois Cochon	Tetragastris balsamifera
Bois D'Amande	Hieronyma caribaea
Bolivian coca	Erythroxylon coca
Boy's love (Southern wood)+	Artemisia abrotanum
Brahminical ginseng	Hypoxis aurea
Bright eyes	Vinca rosea
Burdock+	Arctium lappa
Calamus+	Acorus calamus
Caltrops	Tribulus terrestris
Camel grass	Cymbopogon schoenanthus
Camphor+	Cinnamomum camphora
Cape gooseberry	Physalis minima
Cardamon	Ellettaria cardamomum
Carissa	Carissa edulis
Carmbola	Averrhoa carambola
Carrot*	Daucus carota
Cashew*	Anacardium occidentale
Celery*	Apium graveolens
Ceylon sago	Cycas circinalis
Chamomile+	Matricaria chamomilla
Chervil+	Anthriscus cerefolium
Chick peas*	Cicer arietinum
China root	Smilax chinensis
Chinese ginseng+	Panax ginseng

128

Chinese lotus	Nelumbium nucifera
Chinese raspberry	Rubus species
Chinese tea-tree	Lycium chinense
Chocolate*	Theobroma cacao
Chrysanthemum	Chrysanthemum sinense
Cinnamon*	Cinnamomum parthenoxylon
Clary sage+	Salvia sclarea
Cocaine	Erythroxylon coca, E. truxillense
Cockscomb	Celosia argentea
Coco-de-mer	Lodoicea sechellarum
Coffee*	Coffea arabica
Common Plantain+	Plantago major
Common speedwell+	Veronica officinalis
Concombre zombi	Datura stramonium
Coriander*	Coriandrum sativum
Costus	Saussurea lappa
Cotton	Gossypium herbaceum
Cowhage/Cowitch	Mucuna pruriens
Crab's eyes	Abrus prectorius
Cress	Lepidium sativum
Cubebs+	Peper cubeba
Damiana+	Turnera diffusa var. aphrodisiaca
Dammar resin tree	Shorea robusta
Date palm*	Phoenix dactylifera
Dill*	Anethum graveolens
Dodder	Cuscuta species
Double coconut	Lodoicea sechellarum
Durian	Durio zibethinus
Earth nut/Earth almond	Cyperus esculentus
East Indian globe thistle	Sphaeranthus hirtus
East Indian lotus	Nelumbium nucifera
East Indian sage	Salvia plebeia
Eggplant*	Solanum melongena
Ergot	Claviceps purpurea
Ethiopian pepper	Xylopia aethiopica

129

European ash+	Fraxinus excelsior
False Damiana	Chrysactina mexicana
False Pareira Brava	Chasmanthera owariensis
Fennel*	Foeniculum vulgar
Fenugreek+	Trigonella foenum graecum
Field eryngo	Eryngium Campestre
Figwort+	Scrophularia oldhami
Fingerleaf morning glory	Ipomoea digitata
Finocchio/Fennel*	Foeniculum vulgare var. dulce or F. var. azoricum
Flax seed+	Linum usitatissimum
Florence fennel+	Foeniculum vulgare var. dulce or F. var. azoricum
Fragrant screwpine	Pandanus ordoratissimus
Galangal*+	Alpinia galanga
Garden cress	Lepidium sativum
Garden rocket	Eruca sativa
Garden sage+	Salvia officinalis
Garlic*	Allium sativum
Gat	Catha edulis
German chamomile+	Matricaria chamomilla
Ginger*	Zingiber officinale
Ginseng+	Panax
Globe-thistle+	Echinops echinatus
Goat's rue+	Galega officinalis
Grains of Paradise+	Aframomum melegueta
Great ox-eye bean	Mucuna (Stizolobium) giganteum
Ground bread	Cyclamen europaeum
Ground cherry	Physalis angulata
Guinea cubebs	Piper guineense
Guinea pepper	Xylopia aethiopica
Haemorrhage plant	Aspilia latifolia
Hawkweeds	Hieracium species
Heart-leaved moonseed	Cocculus cordifolius

Heart-leaved moonseed	Tinospora cordifolia
Hedge-parsley	Torilis japonica
Hemp (Marijuana)	Cannabis sativa
Herb of Grace (Rue)+	Ruta graveolens
Hog-plum	Spondias lutea
Honeysuckle	Lonicera japonica
Hops+	Humulus lupulus
Horseradish tree*	Moringa oleifera
Iceland moss+	Cetraria islandica
Ignatius beans	Stryhnos ignatii
Indian butter tree	Madhuca latifolia
Indian cup-plant	Silphium perfoliatum
Indian mallow	Abutilon indicum
Indian nightshade	Solanum indicum
Indian orchid	Dendrobium macrael
Jak fruit tree	Artocarpus heterphyllus
Jamaica ginger*	Zingiber officinale
Jasmin	Jasminum grandiflorum
Jequirity	Abrus precatorius
Jumbi seeds	Abrus precatorius
Khat	Catha edulis
Lad's love (Southernwood)+	Artemisia abrotanum
Lady's bed-straw+	Galium luteum
Leane bandee	Rhynchosia phaseolides
Leeks*	Allium porrum
Letter plant	Grammatophyllum speciosum
Lettuce*	Lactuca sativa
Licorice+	Glycyrrhiza glabra
Lipstick Plant*	Bixa orellana
Little pinkie	Vinca rosea
Lotus	Nelumbium
Maerua	Maerua angolensis
Mai-gung/Mak-tung	Ophiopogon japonicus
Mamey	Mammea americana
Mandrake	Mandragora officinarum

Mangosteen species	Garcinia mannii
Mangrove	Avicennia species
Marijuana	Cannabis sativa
Marjoram*	Origanum majorana
Marking nut	Semecarpus anacardium
Masterwort	Imperatoria ostruthium
Mints+	Mentha species
Monk's pepper	Vitex agnus castus
Mullein+	Verbascum Thapsus
Musk melon*	Cucumis melo
Musk-scented rose	Rosa moschata
Mustard*	Brassica alba or nigra
Mustard tree	Salvadore oleoides
Myrtle+	Myrtus communis
Nandina	Nandina domestica
Nettle+	Urtica dioica
Niando	Alchornea floribunda
Nux-vomica tree	Strychnos nux-vomica
Oats*	Avena satina
Okra*	Hibiscus esculentus
Old man	Artemisia abrotanum
Onion*	Allium cepa
Orchid tree	Bauhinia variegata, B. purpurea, B. alba
Oriental cashew nut*	Semecarpus anacardium
Orobanche	Orobanche ammophyla or O. major
Pagoda tree	Ficus religiosa
Papaya*	Carica papaya
Parsley*	Petroselinum hortense
Parsnip*	Pastinaca sativa
Pawpaw/Papaya*	Carica papaya
Peepul	Ficus religiosa
Pega palo	Rhynchosia phaseolides
Periwinkle+	Vinca major, V. rosea

Pine sap	Pinus species
Pistachio/Pistache*	Pistacia vera
Poison hemlock	Circuta maculata, C. maculatum
Poison nut	Strchnos nux-vomica
Potency-wood+	Muira-puama
Prayer seeds	Abrus precatorius
Prince's feathers	Amaranthus polygamus
Purslane	Portulaca oleracea
Quaat/Quat	Catha edulis
Ragged cup+	Silphium perfoliatum
Rocket	Eruca sativa
Rose+	Rosa species
Rue+	Ruta graveolens
Sacred fig tree	Ficus religiosa
Sacred lotus	Nelumbium nucifera
Saffron*	Crocus sativus
Salep+	Orchis morio, O. latifoia, O. maculata, O. mascula
Saltpeter+	Nitre
Sarsaparilla+	Smilax chinensis
Satyrion	Orchis
Saw palmetto+	Serenoa serrulata
Schizandra	Schizandra chinensis
Sea-bean	Mucuna (Stizolobium) giganteum
Sea holly	Eryngium maritimum
Sesame*	Sesamum orientale, S. indicum
Shack-shack	Albizzia lebbeck
Shaggy button weed	Borreria hispida
Siberian motherwort	Leonurus sibiricus
Silk-cotton tree	Bombax malabaricum or B. heptaphylla
Skirret	Sium sisarum
Southernwood+	Artemisia abrotanum

133

Sowbread	Cyclamen europaeum
Spanish fly	Cantharis vesicatoria
Spearmint*	Mentha spicata
Spice tree	Xylopia aethiopica
Spignel	Meum athamanticum
Spiny pigweed	Amaranthus spinosus
Star-grass	Hypoxis aurea
Stinging nettle+	Urtica dioica
Strawberry tomato	Physalis alkekengi
Strychnine tree	Strychnos nux-vomica
Summer savory+	Satureja hortensis
Sweet flag (Calamus)+	Acorus calamus
Sweet indrajao	Wrightia tinctoria
Sweet root (Licorice)+	Glycyrrhiza glabra
Taranjabin	Alhagi maurorum
Toad flax	Linaria vulgaris
Tobacco*	Nicotiana tabacum
Truffles*	Tuber melanosporum, T. aestivum, T. brumale
Turnip*	Brassica rapa
Vanilla*	Vanilla planifolia
Velvet leaf	Chasmanthera owariensis
Vervain+	Verbena officinalis
Walnut*	Jugulans regia
Water chestnut*	Trapa bispinosa
Watercress*	Nasturtium officinale
Water eryngo+	Eryngium aquaticum
West African pepper	Piper guineense
White water-lily	Nymphaea alba
Wild licorice	Abrus precatorius
Willow+	Salix alba
Willow catkins	Salix nigra
Winter cherry	Physalis alkekengi
Winter cherry	Withania somnifera
Witton root	Eulophia campestris

Woman's tongue	Albizzia lebbeck
Wormwood+	Artemisia absinthium
Yerba del sapo	Eryngium comosum
Yellow flowering lotus	Nelumbo lutea
Yellow water-lily	Nelumbo lutea
Yohimbe+	Pansinystalia yohimbe
Zo douvant	Eugenia crenulata
Zombi cucumber	Datura stramonium

GLOSSARY OF UNFAMILIAR TERMS

Antiscorbutic: Cures or prevents scurvy.

Anthelmintic: A remedy which expels worms from the body.

Aperitive [Aperient]: Gently laxative, without purging.

Atony: Lacking tone or nervous energy.

Attenuating [Attenuate]: Slender; thin; reduced to thinness.

Cachectic [Cachexy]: A depraved condition of the body in which nutrition is everywhere defective.

Deobstruent: Removes obstruction, generally by mild laxative effect.

Decoction: A preparation made by pouring cold water on cut, bruised or ground leaves, barks, roots or other parts of the plant. The mixture is boiled for 20 to 30 minutes, then cooled and strained. Decoctions are generally made in a strength of 1 ounce to the pint; but as the water boils off, it is best to use 1-1/2 pint, as the decoction should, when finished, measure 1 pint.

Demulcent: Soothing, mucilaginous; relieves inflammation.

Depurative: Purifies the blood and fluids in the body.

Electuary: A medicine composed of powders, or other ingredients, incorporated with honey or syrup to form a pasty mass.

Emmenagogue: Promotes menstruation.

Farinaceous: Consisting or made of flour or meal; having such an appearance; yielding flour or starch.

Febrifuge: Abates or drives away fever.

Fomentation: Application to the surface of the body of flannels, etc., soaked in hot water, whether simple or medicated, or any other warm, soft medicinal substance.

Hemostatic: Having the property of stopping hemorrhage; styptic.

Infusion: A preparation made of ground or bruised roots, barks, seeds or leaves, by pouring boiling water over the plant, letting it stand for 30 minutes, occasionally stirring and carefully straining off the clear liquid. The usual quantity of herb is 1 ounce to 1 pint of water.

137

Jaggery: In India, a coarse brown sugar made by evaporation from palm sap.

Mucilaginous: Having the nature and properties of mucilage: soft, moist, viscous.

Omphacine: An oily liquid expressed from unripe olives or grapes.

Pectoral: Medicines considered effective for relieving affections of the chest.

Stomachic: Strengthens and gives tone to the stomach; a tonic.

Tincture: A spirituous preparation made with alcohol or spirits of wine for herbs containing gummy, resinous or volatile properties. Herbs rendered useless by the application of heat in any form and those which will not yield their properties to water alone are most often prepared as tinctures. They are better held in spirituous solutions and are better preserved from deterioration. Tinctures are generally made in a strength of 1 or 2 ounces of herb to the pint.